MW01096390

ENDORSEMEN

"As we recognize our _____ holistic relationship w _____ plant-spirit practices. An important and informative book, based on the Seed Sistas' many years of working with these enigmatic and sometimes controversial herbs. Here the plants become our teachers and guides on our journey toward spiritual regeneration, personal transformation and healing our relationship with the Earth. Thank you Seed Sistas; this comprehensive book really adds to my journey!"
Glennie Kindred, herbalist and author

"The Seed Sistas are at it again, spreading the good word of the herb, gathering our gracious green allies and telling their stories so eloquently. I hope this new book travels far out into the world like a wild tenacious seed."
Rosemary Gladstar, herbalist and author

"This is a treasure of a book, full of gems and precious words of wisdom, delving deep into a dark subject and shining light on old practices and traditional knowledge. A textbook, a story book, a book for clinicians and the curious lay reader alike. Engrossing and engaging, with beautiful photographs and illustrations throughout. *Poison Prescriptions* is a feast for the eye as well as a source of important clinical information. I shall be referencing back to this book again and again."
Chanchal Cabrera, Chair of Botanical Medicine, Institute of Naturopathic Medicine

"Plant medicines provide a vital tool to help us reconnect to each other and our wider nature. We need to get beyond our recent fear-driven narratives and remember just how healing and expansive our native plant allies are. This book is a great start to doing just that."
Bruce Parry, TV presenter and indigenous rights advocate

"The Seed Sistas' commitment to seeds, plants and nature is a source of inspiration for us all. Read this amazing book and be informed and inspired. You will discover the magic and mystery of nature."
Satish Kumar, Editor Emeritus, Resurgence & Ecologist magazine and Founder of Schumacher College

"A long overdue book for the current psychedelic era that reaches far back into our witchy European past. The Seed Sistas have once more brewed up a vital grimoire for those wishing to follow the poison path as a means of healing ourselves and our connection to nature."
Dr David Luke, Associate Professor of Psychology, University of Greenwich

"The Seed Sistas bring the essence of earth, magic, mystery and wild beauty to life, weaving grounded wisdom, ancient folklore and practical learning between the pages of this book. They are safe and knowledgeable guides with which to explore the plant allies and their deepest secrets."
Brigit Anna McNeill, forager, herbalist, wild plant medicine teacher

"A true grimoire for working with the spirits of witchcraft, *Poison Prescriptions* provides an accessible introduction to a family of herbs beloved by the occult tradition. In this book's blend of indigenous magical knowledge and modern pharmacology, the Seed Sistas serve up a careful, comprehensive and inspiring re-evaluation of the 'hexing herbs' and provide practical, suitably cautious and transformative ways for readers to engage with these magical medicines."
Julian Vayne, occultist, writer and psychonaut

"This is the book we've all been waiting for; the gifts within are profound and divine. Thank you, Seed Sistas, for your depth of knowledge, your belief, your power as healers and for guiding us to heal our relationship with nature."
Ayana Iyi, The Black Widow, High Crone Warrior Priestess

"Poetic and majestic, wise and wary, this book speaks to us from lifetimes of experience and a deep abiding love for the herbs that live with us. By reading this book, we gain clues to better health, ways of moving through life's trials and a sense of the deep roots of herbal practices in all cultures. "
Nikki Wyrd, editor of the Psychedelic Press Journal *and Director of the Breaking Convention psychedelic conference*

"The wonderful Seed Sistas have created another beautiful book about plants, this time about some of our sacred teachers whose use is largely lost in modern times. Full of fascinating folklore, science and information of all kinds."
Pip Waller, author of Touched by Nature *and* Deeply Holistic

ILLUSTRATED
BY SILVA DE MAJO

THE SEED SISTAS

POWER
PLANT
MEDICINE,
MAGIC
& RITUAL

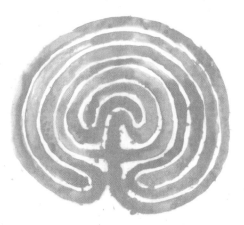

POISON
PRESCRIPTIONS

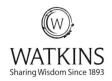

WATKINS
Sharing Wisdom Since 1893

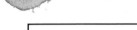

NOTE OF CAUTION

This book intends to educate but does not prescribe treatment for any ailments. Be self-aware, self-respectful and conscious of all risks associated with these powerful plants. Consult with a practitioner before experimenting with herbs (especially if you are taking any medication), be sure to understand herb–drug interactions beforehand and always be extra cautious in pregnancy or while breastfeeding. Please be responsible and hold good intentions in your heart.

The information in this book is not intended as a substitute for professional medical advice and treatment. If you are pregnant or are suffering from any medical conditions or health problems, it is recommended that you consult a medical professional before following any of the advice or practice suggested in this book. Watkins Media Limited, or any other persons who have been involved in working on this publication, cannot accept responsibility for any injuries or damage incurred as a result of following the information, exercises or therapeutic techniques contained in this book.

Poison Prescriptions

The Seed Sistas

Illustrated by Silva de Majo

First published in the UK and USA in 2022 by Watkins, an imprint of Watkins Media Limited
Unit 11, Shepperton House, 83–93 Shepperton Road, London N1 3DF

enquiries@watkinspublishing.com

Design and typography copyright © Watkins Media Limited 2022
Text copyright © The Seed Sistas 2022
Artwork copyright © Silva de Majo 2022
Photography copyright © Seed Sistas 2022

The right of The Seed Sistas to be identified as the authors of this text has been asserted in accordance with the Copyright, Designs and Patents Act of 1988.

All rights reserved. No part of this book may be reproduced in any form or by any electronic or mechanical means, including information storage and retrieval systems, without permission in writing from the publisher, except by a reviewer who may quote brief passages in a review.

Publisher: Fiona Robertson
Assistant Editor: Brittany Willis

Copyeditor: Sue Lascelles
Head of Design: Karen Smith
Design Concept: Francesca Corsini
Designer: Alice Claire Coleman
Commissioned Artwork: Silva de Majo
Photographer of the author portrait on page 304: NUX Photography
Production: Uzma Taj

A CIP record for this book is available from the British Library

ISBN: 978-1-78678-714-9 (Hardback)
ISBN: 978-1-78678-726-2 (eBook)

10 9 8 7 6 5 4 3 2 1

Printed in China

www.watkinspublishing.com

Abbreviations used throughout this book:
CE Common Era (the equivalent of AD)
BCE Before the Common Era (the equivalent of BC)
b. born, d. died

MIX
Paper | Supporting responsible forestry
FSC™ C005748

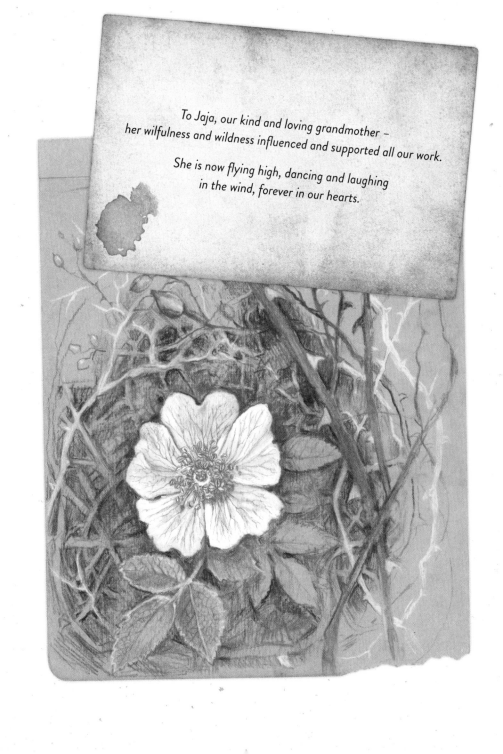

To Jaja, our kind and loving grandmother –
her wilfulness and wildness influenced and supported all our work.

She is now flying high, dancing and laughing
in the wind, forever in our hearts.

CONTENTS

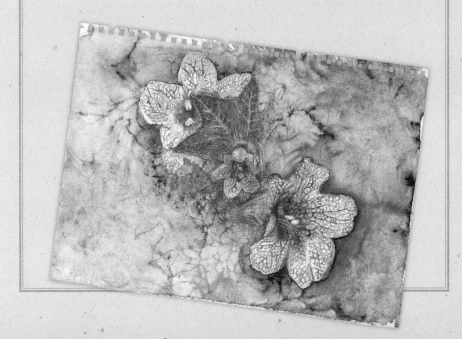

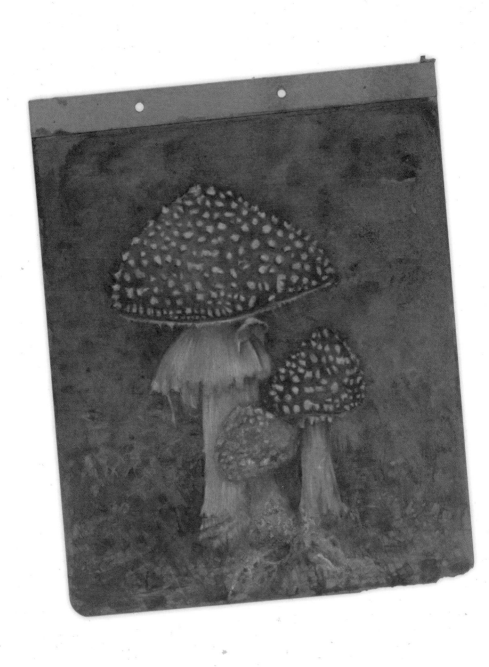

FOREWORD
BY NENEH CHERRY

I am so thrilled that you have found yourself in possession of this special book, which is in itself a little bit of magic, touching on the rediscovery of old ways of being and reintegrating medicine and ritual.

When I was growing up, any cold I caught would travel straight down to my chest and I suffered horribly from chronic bronchitis. Since this is absolutely dreadful for a singer, I sought the aid of witchcraft from one of my vocal teachers early on in my career.

She was a classical singing tutor, and I went to her weekly. In one session I was coughing and she said, "Listen dear, we need to do something about this." She instructed me to bring her some of my hair, which was whisked away to be miraculously tested with a pendulum. This mysterious dowsing led me to discover a wealth of alternative approaches to my own health needs – approaches that have served me well and opened my eyes to the fact that health is not only physical but also has emotional and spiritual aspects.

I first met the Seed Sistas one midsummer at Glastonbury Festival. My bronchitis typically worsens when I am tired and working intensely, so unfortunately it makes an appearance frequently at gigs.

What a godsend the Seed Sistas, with their incredible potions, turned out to be. My daughter took me to meet those witchy women in their funky caravan. Without a pause they knew what I needed and had just the thing; their healing hands and energy instantly made me feel better.

This kind of alchemical therapeutic knowledge is so vital and rare in the modern world. I purchased a remedy they had in stock – something they called Tonsil Tickler. All the herbs were cultivated and cared for from their garden and the remedy was created in their kitchen. I sprayed the elixir into my throat, and miraculously my voice slowly returned and I was able to sing again!

The Seed Sistas are hopeful and brimming with the belief that we can create a more naturally connected world. I fully believe the sentiment and foundations of their work is much needed in the world right now.

I'm flattered to be writing this foreword for such an important work. Poison Prescriptions harnesses a way to start healing ourselves and improve our understanding that we are part of the whole and the cosmos. We are at a specific place and time in this world where feelings of helplessness are rife – this is a time for us to own and understand our own magic and fully possess these enchanting ways. We need to listen carefully to the messages of the cosmos. By craving dialogue with the universe and nature, we find ourselves at a starting point to help one another and ourselves.

I feel inspired by the Seed Sistas. What they've created here motivates and encourages deeper comprehension of the witching herbs, the incredible plants that have the power to heal and to poison, to give second sight and to alter consciousness, to alleviate pain and suffering and to turn us on. These awesome beautiful plants grace the gardens of the Earth and rouse greater connection with all of life.

May you find the inspiration and connection with nature you are looking for in these pages.

Neneh Cherry

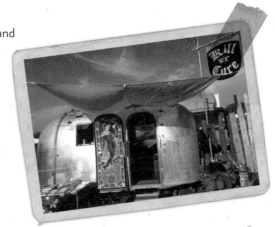

WELCOME TO THE
WITCHING HERBS

 ake yourself comfortable as we welcome you with open hearts to our story of the witching herbs, also known as power plants. We have selected three of our dearest plants that have long been associated with the darker and more mysterious arts: henbane, datura (we're referring specifically to our friend *Datura stramonium*) and belladonna. They are all part of the medical herbalist's *Materia medica*, yet have become scarcely used through lack of education and the fears that surround them. Here, we open a doorway into some of the forgotten herbal magical traditions, shining a light on a shady subject and offering access to deeply hidden spaces. We offer practical magic, spell-work, astrological influences, history, story and medicine.

We hope the wisdom in this grimoire assists you on your journey of discovery in the plant mysteries. Let these words and images support a deepening love for our shared Earth. Watch as the seeds of that love root, grow and flourish. Through nurturing an understanding of the power plants, you will gain intimate access to their long-forgotten history and potential.

Let us begin by asking our polka-dotted friend, the fly agaric toadstool, to interweave connective mycelial threads throughout this book, and, with each spore scattered to the winds, carry the message calling for the reintegration of medicine and magic. We call for a revival of the old ways and for the witching herbs to be reincorporated into the practice of modern herbal medicine and contemporary magic.

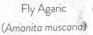

Fly Agaric
(*Amanita muscaria*)

OUR MAGICAL INTENTION

Within this book there is an intention woven into every word; a spell cast to proliferate ancient knowledge, to support trust and to offer security for the practitioners of this cunning craft. Abundance and protection are offered for this work, calling forth respect and reverence, revelry and irreverence for the mysteries of our native power plants, the witching herbs.

The spell sewn into the fabric of this book is an invitation to delve deep into the world of magical plants and to play a part in the reintegration of medicine and magic. We wish for strands of knowledge to embed into you, dear reader, inspiring you to create a healthy relationship with some of the witching herbs described in these pages.

We have written this book to support the changes that are afoot. Today, it is understood that our internal microbiome reflects that of the soil around us and that wherever we originate from or live, there is much to be learned from the plants that populate our local surroundings and grow in our gardens, parks and waysides. We cordially invite you to join us in this work of love and magic.

Throughout these pages, we mention the importance of intention in magical work. When we create our much-loved remedies, one of the key aspects is setting our magical intention – for where attention goes, energy flows.

Intention is the foundation of any magical practice and, as you will see, when working with plants it starts with the very act of growing these beauties, especially when working with powerful healing and potentially poisonous plants.

OUR MISSION

We are the Seed Sistas, clinical herbalists, wild and wicked witches of the fields, gardens and hedgerows and the tech-webisphere. Sensory Solutions Herbal Evolution is our social enterprise, a vast coven bustling with a community of Earth lovers, each one motivated to inspire others through sharing herbal wisdom.

We both feel lucky to have always had the sense that nature is alive and can deliver messages to us that will guide us, bring us strength and courage, and help us to make decisions in life. We were exposed to the wilds of nature from our earliest years and given the freedom to explore them. It is because of this experience that we have been able to meet the plants in a magical sphere and share our knowledge of them. We have seen misconceptions of the poisons arise over the years, in particular regarding the witching herbs, the nightshade family of plants. We have set out to counter these misconceptions by creating profiles of their healing capacities to help us understand and be guided by each plant's unique spirits.

Nature expresses vibrations and initiates responses, indicating that everything forms part of the universal connection of living things. We know the plants hold a vital spirit; they are sentient beings. They possess souls – also referred to as spirits – which are living entities with volition, moods and the capacity to help or wreak havoc as they are wooed or offended. There is an exquisite uniqueness to each individual soul. With the witching herbs in particular, we hear their callings and songs. The energy that comes from working magically with these revered plants is essential to our herbalism.

Throughout our lives we have allowed the plants to lead our work and have followed the signs that they have gifted us. As we opened up our hearts and souls to the witching ways, henbane turned up, self-seeded in a pot outside our front door and growing from the rubble on the land next to where we lived. Datura filled the tool yard at a place where we gardened – a beautiful, deep purple variety that we've not seen since. Then we were gifted a mandrake at an event. One night, on a full moon, we found a huge belladonna plant growing between the cracks on the steps of a cathedral in Spain. We felt that nature had granted us access to another sphere of existence; a curtain had been drawn back and we glimpsed a state of being that was out of the ordinary.

It was vital for us to follow the signs and work more deeply with these plants. The more we worked with them, the more they appeared in our lives. We began growing them and researching their history, medicine and magic. By forming friendships with each of our native power plants, we discovered that these potent plants possess such a forceful nature that even just growing them is often enough to alter conscious reality. There is no need to use frighteningly large doses; including them in rituals even in tiny amounts can be extremely potent. We have come to love including the nightshades in both our clinical and spiritual practices. They have enabled us to bring the magic back into the clinical setting.

The witching herbs have, on the whole, fallen out of fashion in the modern Western herbalist's tool kit, which means losing out on some extremely potent and life-enhancing medicine. All too often, modern clinical herbalism has been guided by a wish for its practitioners to be regarded as professionals, akin to doctors. Indeed, our comprehensive university training saw us in a hospital setting, complete with white coats and stethoscopes. While we learned detailed diagnostic and laboratory skills during our studies, the lack of reverence for the spirit and magic of nature left a palpable void.

We believe, as plant lovers, herbalists and healthcare professionals, that we need to rebuild relationships with the witching herbs. We aim to integrate a more receptive, less linear approach to both research into and spiritual practice with these valuable and beautiful plants. That is not to say that more analytical and measurable methods are obsolete, but that we could achieve a more balanced perspective when coupled with the revival of some ancient practices. We believe that these special herbs hold the key to a remerging of medicine and magic. While the physical medicine of these plants is obvious and well documented, the magic and power they bring cannot be denied any longer.

Naturally drawn to delving into the preparations attributed to witches of old, the myth of the flying ointment became fascinating to us – a concoction seemingly lost in the annals of time. Indeed, much of the past 20 years has seen us exploring the history and potential uses of the flying ointments of European witchcraft, which are made from *Solanaceae* (Latin name of the nightshade plant family) plant preparations. We refer to it as a myth because information is scant, and it is hard to establish credibility.

We have scoured the history books and contacted contemporary medical herbalists, as well as witches, magicians and travellers to the astral sphere (such as psychonauts). Our nights are often spent travelling into the dreaming space where conscious awareness has given way to incredible realms. Through studying the European history of the witching herbs, we learned that the cultural framing

of the plants used in the flying ointment as "deadly"
and "evil" has created veils of fear and mystery that
still surround them today. Now it's time to change
the dominant narrative around these plants and
their use in magic.

THE NATURE OF MAGIC

This book is a tool to aid in the practice of
Earth magic, or natural magic. For us, magic
is a driving force of synchronicities, opportunities and
even challenges. It can seem miraculous, a power that creates experiences
outside of the mundane perimeters of life. It can help us to initiate change
through listening to and uniting with the natural power of the Universe and
the energies that flow through all life. When we say "listening", we mean
tuning in to our surroundings with our whole body, with every cell, with every
memory, with every emotional response and thought.

The truth is that magic and the imagination are woven together. Imagination
and wonder are key ingredients in spellcraft, essential for magic to occur, while
energy is what glues the whole kit and caboodle together. Directing energy
through the use of magical intention can create fantastical transformations.

Magic is an art form, and by introducing herbs into your magical practice,
another layer is added to this ancient craft. So it's time to start listening
to the wild whispers contained within plant life, especially the so-called
witching herbs.

WORKING WITH THE WITCHING HERBS

The "Power Plants" or "Witching Herbs" – also known as the "Poisons" –
encourage a re-wilding of the psyche. We humans share a common ancestry
with plants, having evolved together over the millennia. We have receptor
cells in our bodies that communicate directly with chemical constituents
contained within plants. Today, modern science is proving what seemingly
"far out" folk have been talking about for decades: plants can communicate

13

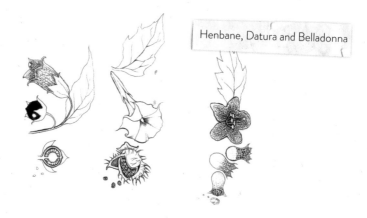

both with each other and with people. They can also learn quickly from experience and adapt to stimuli in their environments.

All plants hold mysteries and stories, each one of them. For example, healing plants have the ability to shift our perceptions when we work with them. However, some more than others unlock hidden, possibly innate knowledge and reveal the secrets of the world around us. In learning to listen to the particularly potent messages of the more mysterious plants, there is a possibility that we can co-create a more balanced medical paradigm and honour the healing experience that they offer. Plants that work to alter consciousness cannot, at this stage, be entirely understood by modern medicine. Herein lies the beauty. We have to suspend belief to a certain degree to work in the sphere of altered consciousness and engage the power of our imagination.

As mentioned in the cautionary note at the start of this book, the witching herbs are very strong psychotropics – potential poisons that can bring on strong hallucinations when taken in larger doses. We do not work with them in this way, nor do we advocate others to do so. We work with them on much more subtle levels, such as by growing these wonderful allies and adding them to our balms, using only relatively minute doses. We are much more interested in the energetics of these herbs and how we can use them to support and promote healthy lifestyles and relationships, both with our own kind and with the plants themselves.

PLANT MAGIC AND YOU

This book is written for anyone who feels a calling to the feral and who is interested in the revival of forgotten knowledge. It is for those of us who want to restore the wild traditions – to be touched by the sacred power plants and fungi of our lands. It is for those who sense the existence of other realms and who wish to learn to trust their intuition and be guided by the plants. And it is for those of us who want practical tools for working with the forgotten gifts of the otherworld and who wish to explore a new paradigm around altered states of consciousness and health.

This book is, at its heart, a celebration of some of the most feared plants of the nightshade family: henbane, datura and belladonna. However, no stars shine alone and we include a supportive cast of other herbs that have inspired us along the way and become an important part of our preparations and spells.

As these words have found their way to you, it is likely that you already have a sense that we are not entirely separate from nature – that nature is not just pretty decoration. Nature is not simply designed for us to observe and look at; it is something we are part of. We are nature. We all are born into this world with sheer wonderment, in awe of the green magic of nature if given the opportunity to experience it. However, our lives can lead us to feel disconnected from the green world around us.

When strengthening your connection with plants, a good starting point is to explore your local wild spaces, gardens and parks. Go plant hunting. In addition to reading this book, get a reliable plant identification guide and perhaps choose one plant and ask to be introduced to it. Take a walk and see what you discover – and don't ignore anything that comes to you on these wanderings, as nothing is linear in this interlaced world of magic. It may take moons of exploration and searching, but so much may be uncovered in this spiral of adventure.

THE LANDSCAPE OF THIS BOOK

Plant ritual, plant ceremony and plant magic are ingrained and intertwined with plant medicine. Our intention is to lead you on a journey through the parks and waysides into the wild, secret spaces of our lands. As a map of the terrain that we will be covering, this book is structured in three parts:

PART I: THE PATH OF POISONS

In Part I, we will explore the history of the witching herbs and why we humans have always been fascinated by altered states of consciousness. We will look at how these relate to magical work as well as personal development, and why witchcraft and the herbs are often given a bad press today. Then we will briefly consider witchcraft around the world, and introduce you to the art of Sensory Herbalism, before touching lightly on the subject of hexes, where you will find

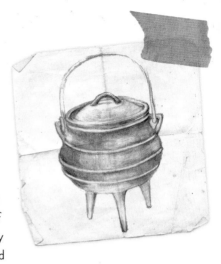

ideas for creating sacred spaces and magical protection. Finally, we will discover the importance of cosmic influences such as the planets and astrological signs, and how these can greatly enhance our magical work with the witching herbs. In particular, we will be focusing on the importance of the moon.

PART II: CONNECTING TO THE WITCHING HERBS

The second part of our story takes us to the stars of the show: the power plants themselves. We will focus on three of the witching herbs that are especially steeped in magic, mythology and medicine: henbane, datura and

belladonna. Looking at the context, importance and reasons why these herbs have been so influential, we will look at each herb individually and explore the profound ways in which they can be used in clinical and personal practice. Finally, we will offer tips and tools to help you connect with the plant world on many levels, such as by creating your own grimoire, storytelling and spellcraft – and discuss how you can get to know plants through cultivating your own witch's garden.

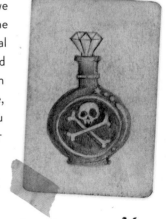

PART III: THE FLYING OINTMENT

The final part of the book opens the doorway to one of our most treasured potions: the flying ointment. Infamous throughout history, we can see how it can be revived today for medicinal and magical practices. Looking at how this potent brew has developed through the centuries, we will share our studies into the ointment and a recipe we have been replicating for many moons, which can help us fly with the support of 13 wonderful plants. We will also be discovering the passion potion and its role in sacred sexuality, and how to use both the ointment and the potion in a range of practices such as divination and trance dancing. Finally, we will consider how power plants within the ointment such as henbane can help us approach death with grace and acceptance.

We recommend that you read the whole book before embarking on any of the practices within it. This will give you a clear understanding of the ways in which we invite you to work with these herbs.

As you plunge into these pages, you will discover new perceptions of sacred sexuality, dream work, death walking, spell-casting and meditative magic. The chapters are full of different ways to connect with the witch or magician within and the green world around. We invite you to explore the witch's medicine cabinet, make magical tools, learn how to create spells and make magic. As you work your way through each chapter, you will glean insights into the forces of an archaic realm that is tapping on your shoulder and asking for your recognition and respect.

We are keen to support your use of witching herbs on an energetic or subtle level, and to dispel any fears and myths that might hold you stuck in a place of self-doubt. We will share our secrets, hopes and dreams of a more connected and compassionate society, with applications and exercises for you to explore on your own therapeutic journey, rebuilding and restoring any fractures or schisms you wish to soothe and bridge.

And now it is time for us to begin.

 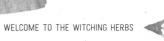

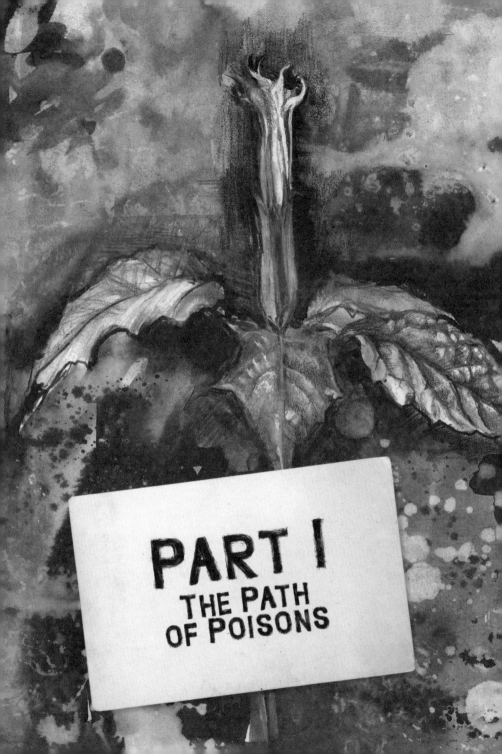

PART I
THE PATH OF POISONS

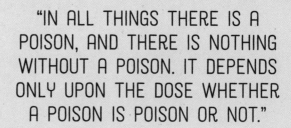

"IN ALL THINGS THERE IS A
POISON, AND THERE IS NOTHING
WITHOUT A POISON. IT DEPENDS
ONLY UPON THE DOSE WHETHER
A POISON IS POISON OR NOT."

PARACELSUS, SWISS PHYSICIAN AND PHILOSOPHER (1493-1541)

Here in Part I, we are introduced to the history of
the witching herbs and, specifically, their relationship
with altered states of consciousness. We will walk
the path of the poisons and explore attitudes toward
witchcraft, past and present, around the world.
We will discover how the witching herbs relate to
astrological influences, and how we can use these
correspondences in our craft for added potency.

- 1 -
POWER PLANTS, POISONS
AND ALTERED STATES

ll herbs hold medicinal gifts and all plants are teachers with the ability to alter our consciousness in some way. We touched on this in the introduction, but you might be asking yourself what we actually mean. Even the most seemingly innocuous herbal combinations can have profound effects in the right environment; for example, we've seen people dance for hours in ecstatic bliss having simply taken drops of elderflower and plantain together. This does partly relate to the individual's ability to tap in to the subtle nature of herbs – and the more you work with them, the more this sensitivity improves to any medicinal herb that you encounter. You learn to observe what is happening in the body and any subtle shifts that may be occurring.

There is no absolute hierarchy whereby one plant is ranked as more important than another. Yet some definitely shout louder to us humans, exerting stronger physical, psychological and spiritual effects on us. These herbs have a greater ability to transport us to other realms and to open pathways, both ancient and new. When used with care and attention, these plants are potent enough to elicit massive shifts in perception, bringing about positive health changes both on an individual and societal scale.

These herbs, the strident ones, are the ones that we will be referring to as the "witching herbs" or "poisons" in this book. They are part of a wider group of plants and plant combinations that have in recent years been labelled "power plants". Some of them have been known about for centuries and have a long lineage of use, although methods have changed in recent years due to worldwide demand. Although there are reported cases of adverse reactions and injury while under their influence, and they can leave lasting emotional damage if not approached with care and adequate after-support, many of them are regarded as being relatively physically safe to use. Ayahuasca (a combination of plants) and magic mushrooms can be considered part of this group. In contrast, the witching herbs are considered by many to be potentially physically unsafe. These herbs are also the ones that have a broken lineage of common use and in larger doses can have unpredictable effects.

Apprehension remains prevalent around these witching herbs of power, as acceptance of unpredictable or unmeasurable outcomes is not generally encouraged in Western society. Misinterpretation of them is therefore rife. Much of what little information remains about them consists of annotations gleaned from the witch trials of the Inquisition (a powerful office set up within the Catholic Church to root out and punish heresy throughout Europe and the Americas), when recipes would have been gathered under duress. This was a horrific time in history when just growing plants such as henbane or belladonna in your medicine garden could have been dangerous. With the subsequent lack of information available, there became the potential of losing the true knowledge from the past.

All of these powerful plants need to be approached with respect and understanding if we are to engage with them. Their effects can be insightful and profound; it would be difficult to ignore the experiences and tutoring that they can offer. They can teach us a multitude of lessons and show us that we are not separate from nature; we are part of it. These beauties open secret doorways into magic.

Magical practices and traditions develop in response to people's surrounding flora, fauna and physical environment. The essence of each plant holds in its energetic body the experiences of those people and places that have gone before – a resonance of the past. This means that it is possible to recreate a picture of ancient rituals through working with and being inspired by our local plants. Yet much has been lost through the neglect of ritual itself in our modern society – ritual that enables connection beyond the self, and helps us to realize that we

POWER PLANTS, POISONS AND ALTERED STATES

thrive as part of a collective. With the help of plants that alter the everyday conscious patterns that we exist in, ritual can take us beyond our individualist nature and create a sense of community. We can then flavour this with our contemporary knowledge and the current circumstances in which we now live. Connecting with these plants of power can help deepen the understanding of what is currently needed for ourselves, our communities and local environment.

Be Conscientious About the Plants You Use

Life is very different in our modern era to anything that has gone before. Access to plants is much easier, as is information about them, with the existence of books, magazines, travel and of course apps and the worldwide web. This presents the potential to be misled by the vast array of information at our fingertips. Intense marketing of psychotropic "experiences" can complicate our motives and can distort a sense of our own place in the world of plants.

When undergoing any work with plants, be supported and guided by people you trust, be discerning about your choices, and feel free to ask questions. Promise yourself that during your explorations you will be conscientious about what plants you take, where they have been sourced and how and by whom.

If taking part in medicine circles and shamanic workshops and retreats, questions to think about include:

* Where did the plant medicines grow?
* Are they wild harvested?
* Who harvested them?
* Are they cultivated and, if so, who grew them?
* Who created the medicinal preparations?
* Do you know what those herbs look like when they are growing?

If the answers are unclear for any of these questions, we would suggest getting connected to the source – the plants themselves. We will talk about the growing plants in Chapter 4 and about the three individual witching herbs in Chapters 6 to 8. This is a route to personal knowledge: trust in your own discernment and find the confidence to ask questions. When you have connected with herbs as they grow, you will start to feel truly connected to nature and emboldened to ask questions of others.

Humans have always walked besides plants, animals and fungi that offer us the route to expanded consciousness through their individual chemical make-up. We have historically enjoyed opportunities to enter other states of being through these other species of life. Compounds within certain plants interact with receptors within our nervous system to initiate these little-understood, altered states. This is evidence enough that we humans and these plants have developed and evolved together; we contain the same compounds and can merge together to experience something beyond the physical self.

All the natural world is full of mysticism. Some plants in particular hold keys to unlocking and awakening pathways in our minds, hearts and souls – pathways that guide us into a multiverse of opportunity and magic.

DOORWAYS TO OTHER WORLDS

There are many reasons why people through the ages have intertwined their existence with powerful plant substances that alter consciousness. Plant ceremonies and rituals have historically been held at auspicious times such as births, puberty, marriages and healing, as well as to mark hunts and death, and to improve psychic abilities. Plants have been used to connect with the divine, to give thanks and to create community cohesion. Many are still in use today, albeit sometimes in different circumstances.

In recent years, for example, substances such as iboga from Africa and toad medicine of the Amazon have been successfully used in addiction therapy. At the time of writing, there are cutting-edge trials in allopathic medicine looking at the use of psilocybin (a naturally occurring psychedelic compound produced by fungi), among other psychoactive agents, to support anxiety and depression. Effects that have been known about since early humans first reached for power plants and fungi are now entering the field of mainstream medicine.

One part of our mission as healers is to educate people around the recreational use of chemical drugs. We wish to see a move away from destructive drugs such as cocaine and heroin. Yet when people move away from more readily available and commonly used drugs such as these, it doesn't necessarily mean that they don't want to experience altered states anymore. Yet with a societal approach of excess, it becomes challenging to apply a more moderated, conscious way to reaching altered states and having connected experiences. People who choose to diverge from familiar but harmful lifestyles often feel isolated when making distinct choices from their peers.

Not only have rituals with exotic psychotropic herbs become commodified in many cases, they can often be extremely prescriptive or even hierarchical, leaving little room for wildness at heart to be fully expressed. There are arguments in support of this approach, in that structure helps to guide and direct the experience, providing an anchor if things get tough while somebody is under the influence of the plant or substance, which is especially valid for those with little experience of powerful psychotropics. However, there is also scope for this attitude to be misinterpreted, as it suggests power needs to be handed over to another authority in order for us to have these experiences.

There is a balance to be struck here. If we are equipped with the knowledge and support we need – and adopt good, balanced practices using fairly traded, responsibly transported and consciously nourishing means – we may find personal fulfilment and enjoyment when experiencing altered states of consciousness. Delving into the sphere of altered states of consciousness in this way gifts us with alternative ways to craft a more inclusive, warm, loving society; it also empowers us to revive playfulness and magic, and indeed investigate a whole new paradigm for medicine.

PSYCHEDELIC MEDICINE

There has been a huge resurgence of scientific interest in power plants over the past 20 years or so. It's a wonderful area of modern medicine that deals directly with all of the unknowns that surround the inclusion of psychedelic medicine in healthcare. The positive effects of psilocybin have been demonstrated in clinical settings, but there is still relatively little understood about exactly how states of altered consciousness are generated. While modern medical science now accepts the therapeutic value of psilocybin, it also acknowledges that many of the mechanisms and effects are currently scientifically unexplainable.

Much of modern medicine remains mechanistic; it relies on putting things into boxes in order to understand, define and categorize them. However, with the incorporation of psychedelic therapies into the field of modern medicine, something very special is happening: it seems that in addition to relying on predictable outcomes, medicine is increasingly prepared to enter the labyrinth and draw on the unknown. Of course, these experiments and therapies are conducted in a controlled way with measurable outcomes!

When British psychiatrist Humphry Osmon first coined the word "psychedelic" in the 1950s, he based it on the Greek word for "mind-manifesting". Over the decades of ethnobotanical and psychedelic plant research, it has been replaced by a stream of other words that have come in and out of fashion. One of these was the term "entheogen", thought up in 1979 by a group of ethnobotanists and scholars of mythology. *Entheos* is Greek for "full of the god, inspired, possessed", and is the root of the English word "enthusiasm", while "gen" comes from *genesis* – to create. This description seems more fitting and less specific when referring to the vast array of experiences that can be created when utilizing plants for magic, ritual and connection. They can indeed induce a feeling of connection to the divine, ideas and aspirations, or, on the flipside, a sensation of being possessed!

The term "hallucinogen" denotes substances that will induce hallucinations. This may be true of many of the witching herbs we will look at in this book, but – as we hope will already be clear – we are not suggesting that they be taken in doses that would induce this state. Nor do we think the common understanding of the word "hallucination" is strictly accurate. It is defined in the Oxford English Dictionary as "an experience involving the apparent perception of something not present". This is a narrow and biased definition of altered states of consciousness, which we personally reject, for it results from our society's cultural disconnect from ancient magical practices. We believe that hallucinations can be perceived as messages for healing from Spirit, and those who receive them may be regarded as lucky or even revered.

As you will have noticed by now, we often refer to power plants as "psychotropics". The word "psycho" (which also relates to being psychotic) has had bad press but originates from the Greek terms *psykho*, meaning "mind, mental; spirit, unconscious", and *psykhē*, denoting the soul or spirit, the invisible animating principle or entity which occupies and directs the physical body. So "psychotropic" means bringing forth the soul and the unconscious, and is a word that closely links to the way we encourage you to connect with these plants.

LEARNING FROM THE POISONS

As we have seen, henbane, datura and belladonna are included among the group of herbs that are referred to as the witching herbs or the poisons. These baneful herbs draw many to them in fascination and trepidation, in the spirit of seeking knowledge and connection with mystery. Long associated with touching the mystical, the *path of the poisons* aids in unlocking hidden entrances, encouraging courage and opening novel avenues for exploration.

Poisons are usually defined as substances that are capable of causing the illness or death of a living organism when introduced to it or absorbed by it. To paraphrase the words of Paracelsus, quoted earlier, everything has the potential to be a poison, for there is nothing without poisonous qualities. It is only the dose that determines whether or not something is toxic. However, there is a much smaller margin of error between a medicinal dose, a psychotropic dose or a toxic dose of our three Solanaceae, or nightshades, than when working with other plants. An informed understanding of any of these plants with a

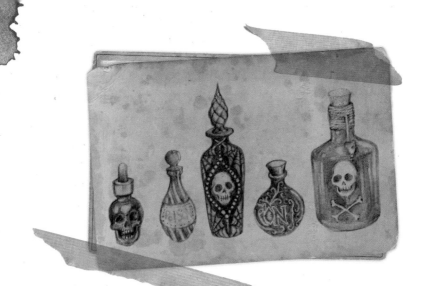

narrower poison margin is therefore essential when creating and taking those medicines and potions that use them. This is why walking the path of the poisons is cultivated over many moons and must be deeply understood on an individual level before administering treatments to anyone else.

Confidence, respect and understanding are needed when using these magical substances. Their potential toxicity is what makes them such valuable medicines. The compounds are extremely powerful. For clinical herbalists like us, these plants provide strong physical medicine, yet today these herbs are little understood and are in danger of dying out of our medicinal consciousness. We have been documenting, gathering knowledge from our peers and working closely with these herbs, reviving their cultivation and deepening our medical understanding of them, developing medical preparations for both subtle, internal physiological shifts and powerful external changes. With their ability to poison, and in most extreme cases cause death, these herbs deserve and indeed command the upmost respect. Demonization and fear are enemies of education and connection, so we counsel careful and slow observations of all these commanding medicinal poisonous herbs – which have been familiar to many down the millennia.

A Short History of the Poisons

The witching herbs have long been associated with power and poison. The term *venefica* means "a female who poisons" in Latin, and referred to a Roman sorceress who used drugs, potions and poison. The path of the poisons is itself synonymous with the art of *veneficium*, referring to the creation of a substance that, when imbibed, alters a person's nature in some way. This medicament, potion or poison can be formed through magic, witchcraft, sorcery or enchantment. It's the place at which poisoning, medicine and magic meet.

Many famous instances of *veneficium* have been noted throughout history. In Homer's epic poem *The Odyssey*, written in approximately the 8th century BCE, datura has been indicated as the plant used in the mass poisoning on Odysseus' ship, when the crew was driven mad. Odysseus managed to avoid the poisoning with an antidote referred to as "moli", which is a name that relates to the snowdrop (*Galanthus nivalis*). (See page 112)

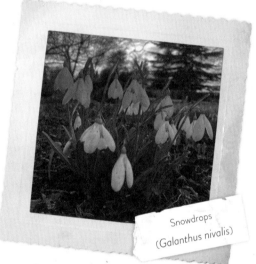

Snowdrops
(*Galanthus nivalis*)

Around 50 CE, the Roman empress Agrippina the Younger requested the services of the infamous Locusta, who had already been imprisoned for poisoning. Agrippina wanted to murder her husband, Claudius, and asked Locusta to supply the poison. Belladonna was supposedly used in this instance. Locusta was apparently loved by Nero, Agripinna's son, who later employed her skills to murder his rivals to the throne. A useful ally for an emperor.

The late 16th-century English herbalist John Gerard referred to deadly nightshade as "Solanum" or "Sleepy Nightshade" in his herbal, where he also talks of the poisonings he witnessed. He warned his readers "to banish these pernicious plants from ... gardens. Otherwise," he notes, "women and children will lust after the shining black berries which are so beautiful." He concludes that the berries are "vile and filthie". What a strange way to write about plants, women and children.

In the 17th century, Catherine Monvoisin, known as "La Voisin", led an organized association of poisoners in Paris. This infamous network provided poisons, aphrodisiacs and abortions, among other practices. They were employed by high-flying figures of the French aristocracy and were said to have killed thousands of people. Herbs used by the network included belladonna, foxglove and mandrake.

In the 18th century, Haitian Maroons used poisons in their attacks on plantation owners and their families. They combined bamboo shoots with poisons from the bush as ammunition in their battles. The famed François Mackandal, immortalized on Haitian coins, was a Maroon leader with a vast knowledge of botany and plant poisons, and organized a plot to poison slave owners through the water supplies. His work and that of other Maroon eventually led the Haitian enslaved peoples to victory.

More recently, in 1910, Dr Crippen was an American homeopath and medicine dispenser who obtained hyoscine to poison his wife. He allegedly poisoned her in England, dismembered her body and eloped to Canada with his mistress. He was hung in Pentonville prison in London after being caught when a telegram was sent from Canada to the London police by a suspicious employer. It was thought that the hyoscine was extracted from henbane.

From these examples, we can see the power of the poison plants being wielded for more power: for revenge, for freedom from oppression or more simply for the purpose of running away with your lover. Women have often featured in connection to poisons throughout the ages, suggesting that knowledge of these plants is associated with the feminine. However, their use of power plants – whether for good or for ill – was forced underground by persecution. The stage was set for patriarchy to run amok in the spiritual realm of ordinary lives.

It is time, now, to reclaim the power represented by these herbs, their archetypes and related deities. After all, the witching herbs are associated with the crone archetype, the goddesses Hekate, Atropos and Kali. These herbs all have a connection with the dark times, the winter, madness and death – the wild, feared, empowered woman.

Hekate the Untameable

Heqat or Hekate, the powerful goddess of Nubian and Greek myth, is a paradox, capable of both good and evil. She is known as both the Queen of the Dead and the protector of thresholds. Originally worshipped as the Mother Goddess responsible for the fertility of all, over time she became much maligned. Triple-faced and bearing flaming torches, she is connected with witchcraft, magic, the moon, doorways and creatures of the night such as hell hounds and ghosts.

Dogs, especially puppies, were typically sacrificed to Hekate. Her connection with dogs may be due to the fact that dogs were known to eat the dead if left unburied. The three-headed hound of Hades, Cerberus, may be an earlier form of Hecate. It is important to note that Hecate may in turn be an earlier version of Artemis, who also has three faces, carries a torch and is surrounded by dogs.

The offerings to the goddess were made each month during the night of a new moon. Female sorcerers often appealed to her for aid in their magic and spells, and she also appears on surviving examples of curse tablets.

In his epic *Fasti*, the Roman poet Ovid wrote about Hekate's triple faces watching over three-forked crossroads. She is the guardian of such crossroads, which were often burial sites for folk whose restless spirits were thought to torment villagers after their deaths, such as those who had died by suicide.

Cerberus

NURTURING YOUR RELATIONSHIP WITH THE WITCHING HERBS

Understanding the witching herbs of the Solanaceae, or nightshade family, can lead to great humility, self-understanding and awareness. Once you have been lured into their realm, you're invited to embrace exploration with open-hearted curiosity. As we will discover, the incredible Solanaceae plants have the potential to open up doorways of perception, shift consciousness, illuminate alternate spheres within ourselves and offer powerful medicine.

In the course of our own studies, we discovered that the smaller the dose of these plants the more profound the experience and long-reaching its effects. There is absolutely no need to work with heroic and potentially damaging doses. Using these plants in what might be viewed as micro-doses helps to blow away any terror of toxicity that surrounds them.

These beautiful, medicinal plants, when grown and included in rituals, can bring great insights and wonderful experiences. Cultivating them invites their spirits to enter into our dreams and whisk us up in a whirling waltz of magic. Investigation into the properties of these herbs is exciting when entered into with self-awareness and respect for them. It is completely safe when approached as an exercise in getting to know each plant energetically.

Through the use of these herbs, we can harness the dream-state to discover information about the health of us and others. We can also form strong connections with our tribes, connected through ceremony, common experience and understanding. We can become more conscious and caring human beings, in the knowledge that humanitarian actions and compassionate aims are of paramount importance for all life.

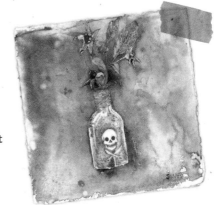

Reciprocity and being conscious of exchange is applied to all our practices with our green friends. What will your gift be to return back to the plant world?

- 2 -
THE RADICAL ROOTS OF MAGIC

 orcerers and witches have existed forever in different cultures around the world, and, of course, still exist today. The qualities associated with them might differ slightly from society to society, but typically witches are maligned and believed to be more active in the dark hours and shady spaces. In the 21st century, there has been a general resurgence in natural medicine and spirituality, animism and witchcraft. Social media in the English-speaking world is full of funky images of pagan practices but, as we will see, witch hunts are still occurring around the planet.

The word "witch" was originally applied to those that were feared – this could have been the cunning folk, the herbalists, midwives or healers. The word "witch" was coined to instil fear in folk about powerful women and recent history has seen a reclaiming of the word as a symbol of power, freedom and knowledge. According to anthropologists and historians, the definition of "witch" then came to mean a person who uses magic to do harm, and was a feared term for the practices of magic and herbalism. So, it was used to create a level of mistrust toward those who understood the natural world and therefore held power within their communities. It was popularized to mean evil or dark. Similarly, the verb "to hex" comes from the Germanic word for witch, *hexe*, and is yet another indication of the historical connection between witches and the act of dabbling in the dark arts for personal or malevolent effect.

Historically, the wise woman has been called upon for her powers, yet also used as a scapegoat to blame for natural disasters such as crop failure or death in childbirth. The edge-walking witch became both feared and revered.

On delving into the history of the word "witch", we came across a reference in the Bible of all places! The Old Testament book of Samuel mentions a sorcerer (1 Samuel 28:3–25). She was in hiding because her powers contravened the law of the land at the time. King Saul had banished all seers and witches from his kingdom – but he then found himself in need of counsel. So he searched for psychic readings to help make decisions about a war he was waging. He had heard of the Witch of Endor and, dressing as a commoner, sought her out. With the gift of her second sight, she of course knew that there was potential danger, so reminded him of the law against practising her art, and gained his promise of protection. They sat in séance and conjured the spirit of the prophet Samuel, who informed Saul that he and his three sons would die in battle the next day and that the Israelites would fall to the Philistines.

The story of the Witch of Endor highlights that ever since biblical times people have been demonized and banished for practising magical arts. The moral persecution of witchcraft reached its peak in Europe during the Early Modern era (from early 16th century), with many nuances as to who, why and for what they were accused. As witch hysteria decreased in Europe, it grew in the Americas during the 17th century, which saw smallpox rip through the land, the French and British warring and constant battles with Native peoples. The most famed of all the witch trials is of course Salem, which took place in 1692, when around 150 people were accused of witchcraft and tortured and 18 people were sentenced to death.

Hostility to witches and magic endured until the 20th century as Western attitudes spread throughout the world with the ships of the Empire. When missionaries encountered the practices of Indigenous cultures, they were often quick to classify these as taboo. Their Christian God brought with Him a defined set of morals and a clear definition of what should be deemed good or evil, and sacred healing practices soon became judged as sinful. European ideals and laws migrated globally during colonial times and seeped into Indigenous beliefs, eroding ancient systems of healing and philosophy. As such, certain forms of magic became synonymous with the Devil's work. We must be mindful that sometimes the very thin distinctions between good and bad expressions of supernatural power are relative and depend on how moral legitimacy is judged.

BELIEFS ABOUT WITCHES

Witch hunts are as old as the idea that it is possible to divorce life from magic.

The ability to accuse one of witchcraft can rock the foundations of a community and in the words of occultist writer Julian Vayne, "that cultural othering and dehumanisation is just as likely to develop top down as bottom up, and that when it emerges from cultural elites that dehumanization can include legal and sometimes lethal force". There were persecutions of many forms: religious, LGBTQ+, single aging women or those with disabilities. It was a horrific and destabilising time.

The history books show that the mass killing of people spread a hysteria; suspicion and unrest amongst communities.

There was a time when people with herb lore stood at the epicentre of every community, consulted about each rite of passage. Often women, they would be turned to for matters of fertility, pregnancy, birth and death. The plants spoke to these women, gifting them with the wisdom of their roots, mycelium, green parts, flowers and seeds.

Many women were feared; their autonomy and sovereignty were not to be left in peace. They were hunted, tortured, killed. In Europe, the practice of witchcraft was considered a crime. Until 1682 in France and 1736 in Britain, practising witchcraft or consulting with a witch was punishable by death. There was a subtle shift in attitude when the new Witchcraft Act was brought in. Rather than punishing folk for witchcraft, the new act actually denied the existence of witchcraft at all. This meant that you were punished for claiming to be a witch or to have contact with the supernatural. The Witchcraft Act lasted well into the 20th century. The last person to be convicted under the Witchcraft Act in England was Jane Rebecca Yorke in late 1944.

Long since outlawed in many parts of the globe, witch hunts continue to pose a problem in parts of Africa and certain (often Christian) communities in the Americas, Asia and Australia. There is still a strong belief that witches are spiteful, wicked creatures who will cause harm through dark magic. Here are just a few examples of how witches are viewed across the globe:

AFRICA

The term "witch doctor" is both broad and controversial, colloquially used to identify traditional African healers. However, this term's root is colonial and anthropologically inaccurate, and its use has historically enforced ridiculously simple stereotypes. Each country and area in Africa has their own indigenous word for the so-called witch doctors, who are usually benevolent healers.

In South Africa, the Witchcraft Suppression Act 3 of 1957 still stands, recognizing acts of witchcraft as illegal.

CARIBBEAN COLONIES

Reforms ended the witch hunts in Europe, but did not include their colonies. The fear that the colonizers would lose their grip on the many lives of their human property was too great. Witchcraft and cultural practices of magic and medicine remained illegal and of course fed into the awful erroneous notion of racial superiority. The late 1700s saw the healing and magical practices of black populations in the French and British colonies become associated with the fear of rebellion and strict legislation was implemented.

CHINA

The label *zhu* is used in some rural parts of China for women who are the head of the household, usually after they have been accused of causing a problem of some sort. These individuals (mainly women) are often ostracized from the community. Families that have *zhu*s tend to stick together and support one another, when support from the wider community would be lacking.

NAVAJO BELIEF

Witchcraft is very much alive within Navajo culture today, existing within a complex spiritual system that includes a dualistic belief in good and evil. The Navaho believe witches to possess a great deal of individual supernatural power; for example, a skinwalker is a type of witch said to travel at night, transforming into the animal whose skin they are wearing. These skinwalkers are said to hold nocturnal meetings, sit among baskets of corpses and use body parts for magic.

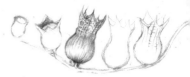

TANZANIA

In Tanzania, attitudes toward magic are accommodating: the majority of rural villages have their own *babu* – a healer who often lives in a hut set away from the community. They are the primary port of call for treating any ailment of the body. Babus are adept herbalists with medical skillsets and vast knowledge of their local plants. Divination is often used as a diagnostic tool, and babus are visited by ancestors or spirits in dreams who aid in creating the medicinal recipes.

RECLAIMING OUR POWER

The oppression of women and herbal lore during the centuries of the European Inquisition, and the subsequent demonizing of the use of the power plants, has partly determined the way that the modern psychotropic experience is sought out today in the UK and parts of Europe. The historical suppression of occult plant use has greatly impacted the way that these powerful plants and the pursuit of altered states of consciousness are approached, even now in the 21st century. The same societal attitudes of consumerism that influence our everyday purchases are applied to trends within the self-help industry and spiritual tourism, including those relating to power plants.

Here in the UK, and across Europe, people book into suburban "shamanistic-style retreats" to imbibe power plant medicines sourced from around the globe. Or do you fancy a Jamaican magic mushroom retreat on a Caribbean beach? We saw one advertised as a "comedy workshop" with bonus psilocybin, a two-week intensive ... What's not to like? Well, whenever you are considering a psychotropic retreat, holiday or escape, there are actually lots of factors to consider – and, honestly, there is plenty "not to like" in the saccharin marketed world of sacred travel. A week on a Caribbean beach drinking mushroom tea with a comedian sounds marvellous to us, but is a very different experience to an Amazonian "plant medicine" jungle escape – or, indeed, to the benefits that come from working knowledgeably with your own local plants.

There is plenty of controversy when it comes to sacred plant retreats and global spiritual tourism. Often, these "healing" and "enlightening" activities border on cultural appropriation. Moreover, the money made from the influx of tourists can divide communities, plants may become over-harvested and there are questions about who is given access to medicines that have been revered locally since time immemorial. This trade can dilute culture, turning traditional healers into little more than guides catering to foreigners. The medicines are no longer about traditions and a community with a shared value system, or about a connection with the elders, but more akin to the patriarchal, capitalist model that we have been trying to move away from in the first place.

Apart from the potentially devastating effects on local communities, there are also issues concerning our own cultural attitudes toward healing. Where whole communities are bonded through shared experiences with plants, you cannot expect to simply step into a "sacred" plant experience while you are there and then re-enter an entirely different societal paradigm on your return. In our experience, one plant or plant concoction, regardless of its potency, cannot be a one-stop cure-all for the heartache, pain, ill health and disappointment accumulated over a lifetime. To turn to a ritual healing and expect all the answers to land in your lap is merely to compound the quick-fix attitude that plagues modern life. In our work, we have often observed people experiencing difficulties in integrating these types of experiences. They arrive home after their weekend retreat or two weeks away and hit the ground running, back to their normal schedule, which misses the opportunity to truly assimilate the healing that has been offered to them. This can lead to further psycho-emotional health issues and, in some cases, isolation. The integration of psychedelic experiences is currently being looked into by certain clinics but is work that is long overdue.

There is obviously a need for better education and information about approaches to healing with plants and in particular the witching herbs, but also the approaches that we generally take toward health, connection and community. Let us focus on building resilient approaches to our health, from the micro to the macro, and look toward an optimistic future that embraces the many facets of treating spiritual, psycho-emotional and planetary ailments. This begins with a literal reconnection to the Earth, getting our fingers into the soil and planting food and medicine. It is a first step toward reclaiming our power and our heritage as self-responsible, wild and connected witches.

BECOMING WILD AND WICKED

Since establishing ourselves as the Seed Sistas, we have embraced the witch archetype, complete with black pointy hats and a cauldron.

At first, we crafted colourful costumes to represent the seasons, and recited stories and poems at festivals, making herbal education the central theme. Requests for love potions and prosperity spells began flowing in, which led us down a new line of research and experience in herbal medicine. Our tiny homes were bursting at the seams with the multitude of tools of the nature-weaver's trade. The walls were lined with shelves of higgledy-piggledy bottles and jars, racks of fragrant herb bunches drying over the stove, bundles of plants hanging from the rafters and countless spiders busy with their webs, brought in with the harvests. Oh, the recipes in our heads that come from our grandmothers, whispered down the generations, keepers of the knowledge, the songlines of old.

When we began taking our homemade herbal remedies out into the world, to markets, fetes and fayres, we soon realized that a huge percentage of the public had no idea what herbal medicine was, let alone that it actually worked. We too found ourselves being both judged and maligned. Our conversations in the plant realms were found to be "freaky" – not part of the conservative world of pure reductionist science.

People would come up to our market stall and challenge us to "prove" the potency and efficacy of the herbs. Our response was to carry research papers about phytotherapy to counter these challenges with clear "proof". We dressed in bright clothing and adorned our hair with blooming fascinators and feathers; our fellow market traders called us the flower girls.

One day at a market in a medieval town square, we found ourselves transported in time, witnessing all the herbalists who had been there before us, plying their wares. In that magical moment the Wild and Wicked

Witches were born. We no longer felt the need to prove ourselves, and we changed our floral outfits for black, blues and silvers. We donned black hats and hung bones outside our herb clinic at festivals, events and on the market.

The Wild and Wicked Witches came about as part of a project to make the more magical aspects of herbalism accessible to those people who might not have otherwise been interested in it. It was also a way of deflecting the challenges we were facing around the value of herbalism. We called what we were doing "Witch Theatre", whereby we embodied the traditional impression of a witch but brought playfulness, story and knowledge about plants to the characters we inhabited, so that people could interact with us and connect with the plant medicines. But issues began to surface with our work. We realized we were alienating a significant section of the public who felt cautious and inhibited around the very word "witch".

We experienced the challenges that women (in particular) have historically faced for being involved in the healing arts. Inevitably conflict of different sorts found us. Some of our peers accused us of not taking herbalism seriously, and there were challenges from the government about the way we were selling our medicines. An extremely uncomfortable time ensued. We had to ask ourselves whether our aim was to enable people to feel comfortable with the word "witch" or to support and open people up to the hedgerow and plant world around them.

In truth, witches still walk these lands, centuries on from the persecutions. Come, walk a while in our garden, taste the herbs, feel the magic, take the power into your own hands. We can all hold this knowledge sacred; open up the spell book, dive in, keep your courage near and your wits about you.

Today, we call the work we practice Sensory Herbalism, because we let our senses lead our discovery of the plants' energetics and personalities – an approach that we wholeheartedly recommend to you. Ours is an emergent tradition, an unfolding of ideas influenced by the past, sensitive to the current landscape and responsive to changes in attitudes and the environment. It is a movement rooted in chaos, ancient yet evolving, influenced by both the whispers of the past and premonitions of the future.

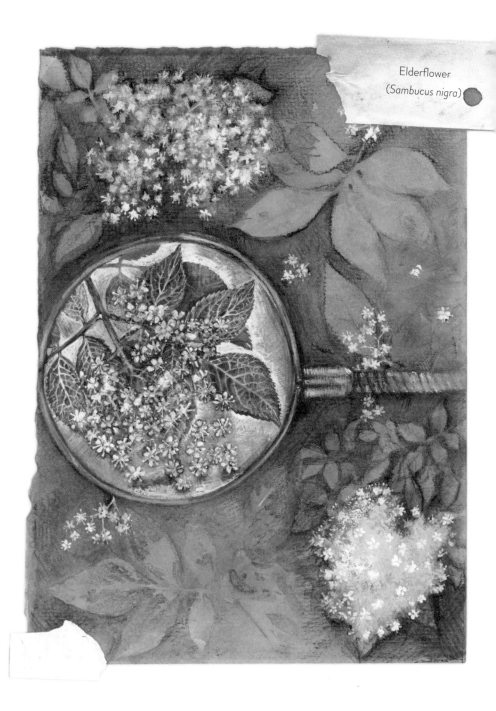

Elderflower
(*Sambucus nigra*)

It is important to us that there is no dogma attached to the work that we do, but instead an opportunity for fluidity and movement. Frameworks can be extremely helpful as a grounding, but they need not remove any power over the decisions you make – and that applies to your work with this book. There must always be room for autonomy, a personal creative flow, to support the development of your herb practice.

NATURE'S SONG

Many people hear nature calling to them. The notes of the song compel them to cultivate a rapport with the plants, and there are a multitude of ways to do so. Attraction to the life-giving energies of plants and trees is a blessing, as is recognizing the awe and inspiration they infuse into our lives. It becomes a caring relationship that runs through all the different aspects of working with plants. Whatever the angle, however people are attracted, we know that the thread of "the love of plants" brings together diverse people and groups, to share and explore their experiences and knowledge, creating a tribe of Earth lovers.

There is a vast scope for plant medicine and plant connection and so many differing careers to choose from: gardeners, botanists, environmentalists, ecologists, ethnobotanists, pharmacologists, aromatherapists, nutritionists, brewers and distillers all have plants at the heart of their work. Plant-craft, herbalism, gardening, sorcery, wizardry and witchery are all art forms as well as sciences. All the Earth's people have an inherent connection to our oldest form of healing: herbalism, the traditional system of medicine.

MALEVOLENT MAGIC

As the Wild and Wicked Witches, we found that along with requests for abundance charms or love spells came requests for us to put hexes on ex-lovers, or to curse competitors, neighbours and work colleagues. It became apparent that there is still a demand for the sort of magic whereby you inflict injury, either emotional or physical, on another.

However, while a person who visits a witch or magician in order to initiate a curse might think that they are handing over the responsibility or karma for the deed, the origin of the maleficence remains with the initiator, even though the witch might be the conduit for the work. The wish for ill-fate comes from the individual, through the energy director.

A curse is usually a form of mal-expression created in a ritual, wishing some sort of adversity or misfortune to befall an individual or entity (this could include a plan, organization or any form of energy that you wish to alter). Greater powers of the spiritual, the gods/goddesses/Spirit and the natural forces are called on to aid in this wish to jinx another.

We do not agree to these requests. In our experience, magic can easily backfire. By drawing attention to that sort of negativity, the individuals who want to hex others are attracting all of that manipulative intention back toward themselves, like an energetic beacon of revenge or malice.

The exception that we make in this book is in Chapter 10 – and that is a curse on wanton consumerism for the benefit of nature, so ultimately intended for the good of the planet.

REMOVAL OF HEXES

People also come to us for the removal of what they feel to be hexes. Interestingly, attitudes toward psycho-emotional illnesses change according to the time or place in which we live. In many places, depression is thought to be the result of spirits or entities attaching to someone and sucking energy from the host. We work with the idea that old connections and links that you feed with your thinking take energy away from current relationships or projects. In this way, severing energetic ties and healing the wounds left behind is essential to good emotional and energetic health.

There is also a whole science of reversal or elimination of these types of curses, where the "spell" has to be "dispelled" through another form of ritual. Middle Eastern and Mediterranean culture has the concept of the "evil eye", perhaps thought to be the effect of envious neighbours and friends, but sometimes the result of a deliberate curse. Protection is gifted by wearing or hanging up a glass effigy of an eye. We choose to bring belladonna into this particular work – her own affinity with eyes is well documented. Her namesake, the Fate Atropos (see page 166), has a sharp pair of shears which are useful to draw on in the cutting of binds to unhelpful energies, freeing us from binds and offering powerful protection too.

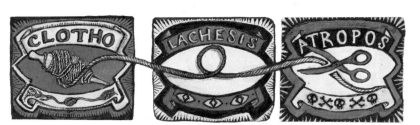

PROTECTION IN MAGICAL WORK

It is a sensible precaution to protect yourself energetically before you start giving away all your magical energy in spellcraft or otherwise leaving yourself vulnerable without considering your emotional or spiritual bodies. After all, the idea of creating protection is not just dogma that has been concocted by practitioners of magical work; it is something that we bring into many different aspects of our lives – for example, we might carry an umbrella in the rain, or put essential oils on our skin to protect ourselves from being bitten by insects.

Plants have naturally developed their own methods of protection from environmental stresses, strains, insects and pathogens. In fact the very alkaloids, that we will go into depth looking at later, are known as secondary metabolites and thought to be created by the plant as protection, making the plants bitter and thus less tasty to predators. Look at nettle and those incredible hypodermic syringe stings; or the black thorn whose lethal spikes are covered in bacteria that can cause skin infections; or the barbed thorns on roses. Strength and safety can also be found in numbers in the plant world, through different growing formations and the size of those barbs; for example, in the superfood-rich, nourishing hedgerow, this is especially true of the cousins of the rose family, such as rosehip, sloe and hawthorn. In human terms, this is reflected in protest movements where people risk their freedom but stand strong and protected together, supported by their fellow comrades.

Following the example of the herbs, we recommend that you protect yourself when opening up to magic, to reduce the potential complications that can arise from giving freely, such as lacking boundaries and allowing energy vampires to take hold. In magic pay attention to how you can take the best measures to achieve your goals while keeping as safe as possible.

When we open up energetically in spellcraft, it is important to stay secure so that our hearts can be open, we can receive any gifts from the Universe and we can move forward with our missions from a place of trust. This is why for your own protection it is good to observe what you imbibe and ingest leading up to the work, cleanse yourself in a ritual bath or shower before you begin and frame the actual work by creating a safe space through "casting a circle".

Cast a Circle for Protection

As you are opening yourself up to all of the elements and subtle energies in spell-work, putting some thought into protection is prudent. We recommend that you begin spell-work by creating a safe space through casting a circle – marking out a circle with intention around yourself. Casting a circle is a bit like walking the boundaries. The physical act of walking around and observing what is around you will prepare your mind for magical work. This can be done using smoke, salt, petals, chalk or, if you wish, by simply imagining a bubble of light surrounding you. Cast a circle when working with any of the magical practices in this book.

Energetic protection during rituals might also take the form of carrying a talisman or lighting incense. A fabulously scented and powerful protective blend of frankincense, angelica root, juniper berries and myrrh can be made into an incense cone, or loose herbs such as mugwort, rosemary, rue and cinnamon can be burned on a charcoal disc. When working with resins and gums from exotic places you should familiarize yourself with their sourced and ethical practises.

For physical protection, think about supporting your liver with the likes of milk thistle. For more information on this, see page 242.

HONEY AND ROSEMARY PROTECTION RITE

*Here is a simple, delicious and effective protection rite
that you can perform whenever you wish to seek a little
extra magical protection for yourself or others.*

You will need:

* a pen and paper
* 1 beeswax candle (or vegan-friendly naturally
  dyed candle to represent bees)
* 1 tsp good-quality local honey (visualize the bees for a vegan alternative)
* 1 red ribbon
* sprigs of rosemary
* 1 homemade flapjack

Steps:

1. Put a date in your diary for your protection rite. Write down exactly
   what you, or whoever you are protecting, need protection from.
2. Light the beeswax candle while saying a few words of gratitude for
   the bees. Take a moment to reflect on their energy and magic.
3. Take a spoonful of honey and taste the sweetness (if
   you are vegan, visualize the bees instead). Ask the bees
   to bring their connectivity and power to this rite.
4. Look at the candle's light and ask the element of fire to surround
   you with its protective glow. Visualize bright, warm light enveloping
   you and radiating out, burning away any negativity or danger.
   Feel the light as a protective armour, keeping you safe.
5. Breathe, filling your lungs with each inhalation
   and fully exhaling for five breaths.

6. Take the ribbon and wrap the rosemary into a bundle with it, taking time to smell the aroma of the herb while repeating:

> I call on you, Rosemary, Rosmarinus, Dew of the Sea,
>
> Please hear my words and protect me [or whomever] from all dangers,
>
> Protect me [or whomever] from harm.

7. Offer thanks to the rosemary, the flame and the bees. You can then imagine the bees pollinating the rosemary.
8. Let yourself feel protected; sit in this feeling of safety and security.
9. Eat your flapjack, then write down any notes or reflection. Then blow out the candle knowing that you have "plugged into the mainframe" and are safe.

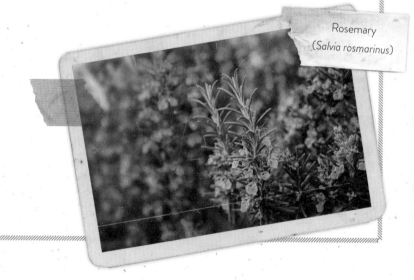

Rosemary
(Salvia rosmarinus)

THE IMPORTANCE OF A SACRED SPACE

When connecting with the Spirit, it helps to have a special ritual space. Such a place for direct communication with divinity can be cleansed and be a place of purity – clear, calming and organized. In this space, the imperfections and deficiencies, the mess of normal life, can be put aside. Like casting a circle, creating a sacred environment helps us to focus on our ritual or intention and therefore protects the work being done.

There are many ways you can recognize or mark that you have considered this aspect of ritual. To begin with, simply designate a special area of your home as your sacred space. You may even like to consider using a screen, curtain or other boundary to make your space feel more contained, relaxing and personal. Get creative and think about colours, fabrics or textures that you love, inviting vibes of relaxation and clarity.

Also set a particular tone for your sacred space; for example, if this is a place for plant magic, you may want to have vases, seeds, roots or potted plants in it. (If using roots, be aware not to dig up wild stock, but instead work from cultivated gardens.) Bring items that have personal meaning and choose objects that give you energy, inspire you or help you get into the meditation, prayer or other sacred practice.

You might find it rewarding to create a regular routine for using your sacred space such as at each full and new moon, setting aside the time for tidying it, sitting in it and lighting candles and offering prayers.

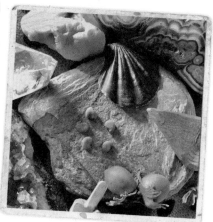

You could also make a special altar in your sacred space for your magical work. Altars are sacred, defined spaces used in wisdom traditions, world religions and in the personal homes of spiritual seekers of all backgrounds, all over the globe – but yours can be personal to you.

CREATING AN ALTAR

Altars are creative, attention- and intention-focusing tools that can be employed to potentiate all your plant magic work. Your altar is somewhere you may go to daily to recharge with positivity, and to gain inspiration for finding moments of release and relaxation, and a place in which to learn more insights about the lovely herbs.

Steps:

1. *Clear a surface in your home and place a few significant objects and plants onto it, for example:*

   * *a photograph of yourself/family/loved ones/ancestors*
   * *your journal or grimoire*
   * *a vase with seasonal flowers*
   * *incense*
   * *representations of the four elements, such as stones (Earth), feathers (Air), shells (Water) and candles (Fire)*
   * *a bowl of water or mirror for scrying*
   * *a small bowl of salt for protection and purification*

2. *You can also change the decorations and colour scheme according to the seasons and what energy you want to potentiate your space with.*

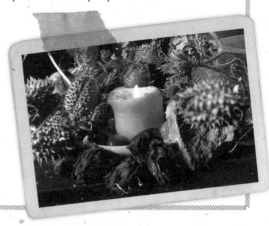

- 3 -
COSMIC INFLUENCES

I t is fascinating to reflect on how life unfolds around auspicious moments. One August night at a gathering of herbalists, we found ourselves in a large patch of blossoming datura, luminescent under a Scorpio full moon. It was as if there were a transference of datura enchantment occurring, encouraging us to follow our hearts and live in accordance with our deepest beliefs. Later that night, we danced passionately to an ever-quickening violin, as the mists gathering over the fields and the moon rose higher. Since that night datura laid out a trail of breadcrumbs for us to follow and the subsequent journey has culminated in the writing of this book.

We have always chosen to follow the signs we are granted and to watch the heavens for information on how best to perform our magic. Thus we try to cultivate, harvest, create our potions and practise magic in line with the cosmic forces as much as possible. The night sky is full of visions and promises.

Astrology is an ancient practice combining science and art, with roots delving back to the Babylonian era. It is far more nuanced than the simple sun signs that we see in the media today, and it has been inextricably linked to plant medicine in many ancient healthcare systems. Applying astrology to your work with plants can provide a framework for understanding them. Through learning about and understanding aspects of the seven astrological bodies of the solar system, including the moon and the sun (known in astrology as the luminaries), and the traits of the astrological signs that relate to these, we instantly have a set of characteristics that can be overlaid on to plants and indeed people.

We tend to simplify the use of astrology in our own work as it can get very complex when linking somebody's natal chart (which maps the position of the celestial bodies at their birth) with their current astrological chart and then layering

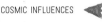

this with their presentation of a disease and its treatment, for example. We also don't work often with the planets that are considered to encompass a generational timescale in their influence such as Uranus, Neptune and Pluto, preferring to work with the luminaries and the personal planets: Sun, Moon, Mercury, Venus, Mars, Jupiter and Saturn. But astrology remains a useful tool on any level.

Choosing the correct moment for seed planting, harvesting, ritual and all magical work by observing our Universe and the cosmic forces at play will suffuse these activities with specific energies. For this, a good astrological diary or calendar is useful.

As you will discover, the witching herbs are themselves associated with particular planets, which can help you decide when might be the best times to work with them and in what capacity.

ASTROLOGICAL CORRESPONDENCES

In astrology, each celestial body is linked to an astrological sign and a particular set of characteristics, some of which are listed in the table on page 51.

In addition to these correspondences, the twelve signs of the zodiac are linked to the four elements of Earth, Air, Fire and Water (see table on page 52). These elements can in turn be expressed as one of the three modalities of cardinal, fixed or mutable.

THE WITCHING HERBS AND THE PLANETS

When reading the rest of this chapter, keep in mind the astrological associations of the individual plants listed below. With time, this information may become second nature to you and inform your work with them.

*   Aconite – Saturn
*   Belladonna – Saturn
*   Datura – Venus or Saturn
*   Henbane – Sun and Saturn
*   Mandrake – Mercury and Saturn

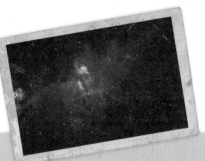

Table of Cosmic Forces
PLANETS OF THE SOLAR SYSTEM

PLANET	ENERGY	ASTROLOGICAL SIGNS
Sun	Vitalism	Leo
Moon	Receptive	Cancer
Mercury	Communication	Gemini Virgo
Venus	Love	Taurus Libra
Mars	Action	Aries Scorpio
Jupiter	Expansion	Pisces Sagittarius
Saturn	Boundaries	Capricorn Aquarius

The personal planets and principal celestial bodies of astrology

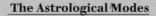

The Astrological Modes

	FIRE	EARTH	AIR	WATER
CARDINAL	Aries	Capricorn	Libra	Cancer
FIXED	Leo	Taurus	Aquarius	Scorpio
MUTABLE	Sagittarius	Virgo	Gemini	Pisces

CARDINAL SIGNS

The energy of the cardinal signs is initiatory. They are like the oldest sibling in the family, and full of the self-initiatory spirit. They assert their particular style of leadership through their element.

FIXED SIGNS

Often thought stubborn, these signs are very driven by their plans to achieve something tangible. They like to flesh out ideas and create form. They will not accept change easily and will need to understand why change is happening and how they can work with and around the change to create conceivable outcomes.

MUTABLE SIGNS

Mutable signs are more flexible. There is a sense of being able to see a situation from many angles, and accept that the only constant is change. They embrace the idea of endings and there is a restless, even chaotic energy to these signs.

THE WITCHING HERBS AND CELESTIAL BODIES

When working with plants, we look at which planets or astrological bodies govern each one. As we have already touched upon, each celestial body has its own qualities. These were assigned to it by early astrologers according to its appearance, what was going on in the world when they were first spotted and various other factors. The planets were then given names relating to gods that best suited their apparent qualities and the influence they exerted over people and plants on Earth.

Are they solid like the Earth or made of gas like Jupiter? How quickly do they orbit the sun? Mercury, for example, orbits the sun in only 88 days and was therefore associated with the quick-witted and fast-paced Greek god Mercury.

Here follows a table listing the planets and a few of their qualities and correspondences, including the witching plants described in these pages. You can use these supportive correspondences when sowing or tending to your plants, or creating potions with them.

The Planets and a Selection of Key Correspondences

Sun

SIGN (AND ELEMENT) Leo (Fire)
QUALITIES Hot and dry, will, aspirations, purpose
BODY Heart and vital force
WEEKDAY Sunday
HERB Henbane, rosemary, hypericum, chilli, daisy

Moon

SIGN (AND ELEMENT) Cancer (Water)
QUALITIES Cold and moist, reflective and receptive, emotions, nurture
BODY Fluids of the body such as lymph
WEEKDAY Monday
HERB Fly agaric

Mercury

SIGN (AND ELEMENT) Gemini (Air), Virgo (Earth)

QUALITIES Moves between types of opposites, such as hot and cold, light and dark; therefore it is none of these principles in itself. Intellect, quick wit, communication, messenger

BODY Nervous system and lungs

WEEKDAY Wednesday

HERB Yarrow, mandrake, fennel, valerian

Venus

SIGN (AND ELEMENT) Taurus (Earth), Libra (Air)

QUALITIES Cold and moist. Love, beauty, attraction

BODY Reproductive organs, senses

WEEKDAY Friday

HERB Mugwort, elder, lady's mantle, rose, marshmallow, foxglove

Mars

SIGN (AND ELEMENT) Aries (Fire), Scorpio (Water) – also ruled by Pluto

QUALITIES Hot and dry, projection, drive, courage

BODY Gallbladder and red blood cells, kidney function

WEEKDAY Tuesday

HERB Milk thistle, chilli

Jupiter

SIGN (AND ELEMENT) Sagittarius (Fire), Pisces
(Water) – also ruled by Neptune
QUALITIES Warm and moist, expansion
BODY Liver and kidneys, physical growth
WEEKDAY Thursday
HERB Henbane, dandelion

Saturn

SIGN (AND ELEMENT) Capricorn (Earth), Aquarius
(Air) – also ruled over by Uranus
QUALITIES Hot and dry, structure, boundaries
BODY Bones, mucous membranes and skin, mineral use in the body
WEEKDAY Saturday
HERB Datura, belladonna

THE WITCHING HERBS AND THE MOON

In addition to understanding their planetary associations, it is particularly important to pay attention to the lunar cycles when working with the witching herbs. The moon affects all life on Earth; it draws the bodies of water toward it, creating tides and flow. As the moon passes through the astrological signs in the heavens, its energy shifts and alters according to the properties of those signs. It therefore pays to be aware of which sign the moon is in and to bring the lunar expression of that sign into any ritual or spell work; working on a full moon in the Fire sign of Aries, for example, may feel very different to working on a full moon in the Water sign of Cancer, as will working on a new moon or waxing or waning moon.

The tides are affected by the gravitational pull of the moon. However, the sun's gravity also affects the tides, accounting for roughly one-third of the phenomenon. When the sun's gravity counteracts the moon's, it leads to lower than average "neap tides". When the sun lines up with the moon, it triggers larger "spring tides". The strongest gravitational effects are felt when the moon and sun pull from the opposite sides of the Earth, when the moon is visible as full. There are also higher than usual tides when the sun and moon are on the same side of the Earth at a new moon.

These same cosmic forces affect the water content of soil, creating more moisture at the time of the new and full moon, encouraging seeds to sprout. Seedlings lie seemingly dormant during their time of gestation before they burst through the dark depths of the soil and reach for the sunlight. This is also true for our dreams, ideas and desires, and we can draw on the lunar cycles to potentiate our individual magic as well as propagate our plants. The dark and new aspects of the moon, with its mysterious unseen forces, offer a nurturing space where our intentions can establish roots before they begin to sprout. The waxing moon encourages the growth of these dreams to come into manifestation at the full moon. As the moon starts to wane, we can use the diminishing light energy to carry away unwanted traits or things that no longer serve us; a banishing can occur.

The Moon's Orbit of the Earth

Our beautiful moon takes approximately 27.5 days to complete one full orbit around our home planet, Earth.

As our moon orbits around Earth, the Earth also moves around the sun. As a result of this double motion, although the moon gets back to its original position 27.5 days later, it takes a couple more days for it to appear as if it is back to its original shape. In other words, while the moon goes round the Earth in 27.5 days, it takes an extra 2 days – 29.5 – to go from new moon to new moon. In effect, the moon has to stretch its cycle by two days to account for the small movement of the Earth around the sun in that time. The Earth is in a slightly different orientation to the sun after nearly a month of travel.

The phases of the moon therefore do not represent one lunar orbit around the Earth. Where the full moon occurs will not always be at the same point on the moon's orbit around the Earth. This is also why lunar and solar eclipses do not occur every lunar month. Sometimes the moon, Earth and sun are aligned, creating eclipses of their light. The phase of the moon is determined by the angle between the sun and the moon as viewed from Earth. The moon can therefore appear as full without the Earth occluding the light of the sun. There are about 12.5 lunar phase cycles in a year.

The moon that we see in the skies above us is awe-inspiring. We can use the orbit of this familiar orb to track cyclical time. The ever-changing movement and shape of the moon give us a framework to support our magical work.

Working with the craft can be viewed as a ritual in itself. The act of cultivating medicines is a long and intricate process. It begins with locating the seeds of the plants, tapping into the lunar cycle to germinate, grow and care for them, and choosing the right astrological time and the optimum weather conditions for the moment of harvest.

You learn the songs of the plants as you work with them, creating their individual medicines, straining or preparing before finally combining herbs to suit the picture or shift that you want to create. There are countless considerations when working with nature. Taking the potions, and using the lotions is the last step of this intricate journey.

THE DARK AND NEW MOON

This is the phase of the moon when there is nothing visible in the night sky. The sun and moon are both on the same side of the Earth. The moon is between the Earth and the sun, so the face of the moon that would be visible to us on Earth is cast into shadow. The point at which the moon is positioned most fully in front of the sun occurs when the moon is at its darkest, but this is also the time marked in a lunar calendar as the new moon. The energy of this lunar darkness can be utilized for this whole period, lasting about a day or two until the first sliver of a new moon is witnessed.

 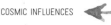

When the moon is fully dark it represents the archetype of the wise crone, the wisdom of the dark. This is a perfect time to create space for introspection, a time to dream, rest and lean into uncomfortable places. You can work with this energy when connecting with ancestral power and if working with hexing energy (which we do not recommend).

During this phase when energies are pulsating in the dark, harvest medicinal roots and rhizomes. There is a sense that the energy is concentrated underground at this time.

New moon is visualized as the time in the cycle when the moon makes her appearance, becoming visible as a thin crescent, a silvery slither, in the sky. This time represents youth and energy. The moon is considered "new" from this moment (around day two of a new cycle) up to the point where the lunar cycle moves beyond the first quarter. The novel, vibrant energies that arise allow magical workings that invite new growth, the start of a project, a chance to start again, creating new beginnings and wishes. The new moon is often referred to as the maiden aspect of the moon. The moon starts to grow or wax in this phase. It is a good time for planting the seeds of your witching herbs.

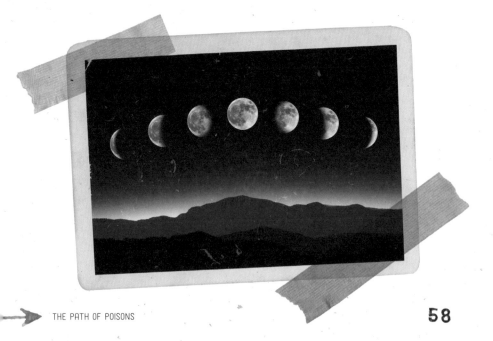

THE WAXING MOON

This refers to the phase where the moon is growing in illumination. It lasts from the first appearance of the crescent slither to the day before the full moon. Observing the waxing moon parallels a sense of growing projects, hopes, dreams, anything that you would like more light directed on. With more light becoming available and sap being drawn up, this is a beneficial time to transplant seedlings.

THE FULL MOON

The full moon is a time of great power, representing generosity and abundance, referred to as the mother aspect of the Goddess. The extended light provides activity in plant growth that occurs above ground. It is the perfect time for harvesting leaves, flowers or fruits. The full moon can add energy to rituals, especially those that need the catalysts of light, power and potency. The full moon is particularly useful for attraction spell-work. It is a time to celebrate successes and accomplishments. It is also an auspicious time for sex and passion magic. Work with sensuality and the celebration of self and confidence at this time. This is an excellent time for harvesting the aerial (above-ground) parts of the plant such as leaves, fruits and bark.

THE WANING MOON

The waning moon is the period from the full moon to the next dark moon. It can be used for banishing work, such as ridding oneself of bad habits or cutting negative influences out of your life. Once identified, these influences can be written down or represented by an object and either buried or burned. We use this time to create a clear awareness around where strong boundaries are needed. Now is a good time to fertilize soil, to weed and prune.

NEW MOON MANIFESTATION RITUAL

Putting aside a few minutes each month during the new moon day(s) to focus on your desires will give you clarity of mind and fill your heart with promise. When it comes to setting goals, there is no better time than at a new moon to start thinking by relaxing into your innermost desires.

Steps:

1. Check a lunar calendar to ensure that it is a new moon and take note of which astrological sign the new moon is transiting through (see pages 62–7). For example, to invite in abundance, choose an earth sign (Taurus, Virgo or Capricorn). To invite passion and drive, work with a fire sign (Aries, Leo or Sagittarius). For clear communication and inspiration, work with an air sign (Aquarius, Gemini or Libra). For emotional understanding, work with a water sign (Pieces, Cancer or Scorpio).

2. Find a moment when you won't be disturbed. Turn off any devices and place a pen and paper nearby before making yourself comfortable.

3. Relax into your breathing, allowing your thoughts to drift. Ask yourself what it is you wish to achieve during this month. Be open to what comes.

4. Now frame those thoughts into an intention, such as "I will … " Write this down and keep it safe.

5. When you are ready, return to your everyday life. Repeat your intention to yourself over the coming days. As the moon begins to grow from the first slice of light in the night sky you can begin to action your aspirations.

6. The moon has its phases and so do our individual wants and needs. This is why it is a good practice to re-dedicate your list of intentions each month when another new moon visits.

THE MOON AND THE SIGNS OF THE ZODIAC

Within magical herbalism, we follow the moon through its various phases and transits through the zodiac in order to enhance the magical and practical work we do with the power plants – from spell-work to growing.

It is good practice to take note of the energetics expressed by the position of the moon during the harvesting of the herbs. For example, herbs gathered while the moon is transiting Gemini will be charged with the energies of communication, and of being quick-witted. This energy will then potentize all magical practices with these herbs, while using a preparation to contain them will bring clarity of communication into the mix.

The luminous sphere that is so mesmeric to us is the closest astral body to our Earth. During its complete orbit from its new to the dark phases, the moon spends around 2.5 days in each of the twelve signs of the zodiac. During these transits there is a sense of the individual energies of each sign being reflected through that of the moon. (For a table listing the plants that correspond with the planetary energies of the signs themselves, see pages 53–5.) We have also added a note for each astrological sign indicating when that particular moon is best for preparing the ingredients of the flying ointment, which we will be exploring in more depth in Part III.

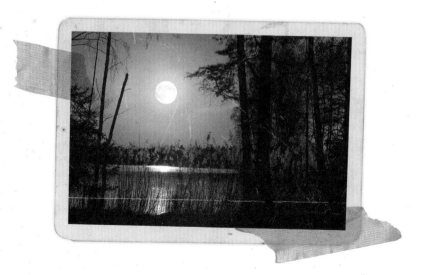

ARIES - THE RAM

* *Mode*: cardinal Fire sign
* *Ruled by*: Mars
* *Key phrase*: "I am"
* *Body parts*: the head, brain and eyes
* *Gifts*: energy, new beginnings, determination, initiation, spontaneity
* *For the flying ointment*: work with belladonna on an Aries moon

The moon in Aries signals a time that is "headstrong". A phase of emotional directness and impulsiveness marked by forceful feelings, with a strong desire to initiate new plans. This is a time to bring determination and drive to magical practices.

TAURUS - THE BULL

* *Mode*: fixed Earth sign
* *Ruled by*: Venus
* *Key phrase*: "I have"
* *Body parts*: neck, vocal cords and thyroid gland
* *Gifts*: endurance, artistry, calm, compassion
* *For the flying ointment*: work with mandrake on a Taurean moon

The moon in Taurus will give a sense of being body-centred and focused on the physical. Feelings of being at peace come into prominence at this time. There may be an inclination to stubbornness and materialism under this lunar influence. This is a time to attract positive energy and a sense of perseverance toward your projects or innermost wants.

GEMINI - THE TWINS

* *Mode*: mutable Air sign
* *Ruled by*: Mercury
* *Key phrase*: "I think"
* *Body parts*: arms, lungs, hands and nervous system
* *Gifts*: communication and connection, multi-tasking, quick-thinking
* *For the flying ointment*: work with fennel and yarrow on a Gemini moon

The moon in Gemini creates an active mind. The instinct at this time is to communicate, think, be inspired and feel light-hearted. The flipside of a Gemini moon is that it can feel restless, changeable and fickle. This is a time to support your nerves or encourage good communication.

CANCER - THE CRAB

* *Mode*: cardinal Water sign
* *Ruled by*: moon
* *Key phrase*: "I feel"
* *Body parts*: chest, breast and stomach
* *Gifts*: a sense of belonging and nurturing, rooting and grounding
* *For the flying ointment*: work with marshmallow on a Cancerian moon

A Cancer moon creates a need for peace and quiet. The need to belong and feel safe permeates this time. This will also feel like a motivational time for putting things in order at home. The moon in Cancer has much healing potential. An insular placement by nature, under this moon placement feelings run deep, making it an ideal time to connect with what motivates you. This is a time to be still and work toward stabilizing energy.

LEO - THE LION

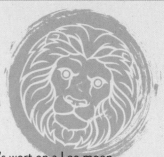

* *Mode*: fixed Fire sign
* *Ruled by*: sun
* *Key phrase*: "I will"
* *Body parts*: heart, spine and upper back
* *Gifts*: romance and creativity
* *For the flying ointment*: work with St John's wort on a Leo moon

A Leo moon is a time of warmth, generosity and whole-hearted loving. However, it can also bring a sense of pride and a feeling of not wanting to fail, which can prevent any emotional vulnerability. This can be a time of attention-seeking, when you want to stand out for your special qualities as well as a strong phase for romance and getting creative. This is a time to bring fire and passion to a project.

VIRGO - THE MAIDEN

* *Mode*: mutable Earth sign
* *Ruled by*: Mercury
* *Key phrase*: "I serve"
* *Body parts*: digestive system, intestines and spleen
* *Gifts*: practicality, problem-solving, making order out of confusion, helping others
* *For the flying ointment*: work with dandelion on a Virgo moon

The moon in Virgo is a good time to find yourself reorganizing and rethinking plans. It has the potential to drive practical solutions, so it is good for getting things accomplished. Health and work goals take precedent under the Virgo moon. This is also a good time to work with plants, gardening and medicine making, as well as to bring a little order to the chaos and to create foundational structures on which to build.

LIBRA - THE SCALES

* *Mode*: cardinal Air sign
* *Ruled by*: Venus
* *Key phrase*: "We are"
* *Body parts*: kidneys, skin, lower back, and buttocks
* *Gifts*: pleasing aesthetics, harmony, balance
* *For the flying ointment*: work with rose on a Libran moon

Creating harmony is the focus when the moon is in Libra. This might appear in different areas such as within romantic relationships. Finding balance may be important at work. Activities that involve self-examination may come to the fore. This is a time to bring beauty and attraction into your work.

SCORPIO - THE SCORPION

* *Mode*: fixed Water sign
* *Ruled by*: Mars and Pluto
* *Key phrase*: "We have"
* *Body parts*: reproductive system and sexual organs
* *Gifts*: sexuality and sensuality, investigation and exploration,
  getting to the "core" of things, creating transformations
* *For the flying ointment*: work with datura on a Scorpio moon

The moon in Scorpio can bring with it intense emotional experiences. This can create a time of deep introspection, exciting new passions or enhanced possessiveness. This can lead to new and exciting appetites or dark brooding and jealousy. Scorpio isn't a light-hearted moon, and could be a perfect time for quiet introspection. The dark atmosphere of this moon phase is an ideal time for connecting with the ancestors. Sit with henbane to provide a portal to this work. The Scorpio moon is definitely a time to tap into your own sexuality and the power and sense of freedom that it can bring.

SAGITTARIUS - THE CENTAUR ARCHER

* *Mode*: mutable Fire sign
* *Ruled by*: Jupiter
* *Key phrase*: "We think"
* *Body parts*: the hips, thighs and liver
* *Gifts*: activity, high energy, adventure
* *For the flying ointment*: work with henbane on a Sagittarian moon

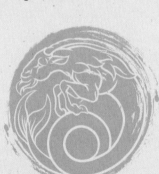

The moon in Sagittarius brings great optimism and positivity, in contrast to the dark energy of the previous Scorpio phase. This moon inspires an expansion of consciousness, travel mentally and also in a physical sense. The desire to journey might be strong in this moon phase and also to learn a new skill or interest. There is seemingly no limit to the sense of freedom at this time. As a result, it is not a good time for decision-making, but instead a time to aim sky-high with planning any projects or ideas.

CAPRICORN - THE SEA-GOAT

* *Mode*: cardinal Earth sign
* *Ruled by*: Saturn
* *Key phrase*: "I achieve"
* *Body parts*: joints and skeletal system
* *Gifts*: trustworthy, connected to the environment and ecology, pragmatic
* *For the flying ointment*: work with dandelion on a Capricorn moon

When the moon is in Capricorn, there is a strong focus on the work aspect of life. It is an ambitious yet practical energy. Creating goals and planning how to get there is a beneficial activity. This is a time to design practical plans.

AQUARIUS - THE WATER CARRIER

* *Mode*: fixed Air sign
* *Ruled by*: Saturn (or in more modern astrology Uranus – Aquarius energy wants to break free from the confines of Saturn rulership)
* *Key phrase*: "We will"
* *Body parts*: ankles and circulatory system
* *Gifts*: freedom, experimentation, thoughts and ideas, progress
* *For the flying ointment*: work with aconite on an Aquarian moon

An Aquarius moon can cause a strong sense of individualism. It is a time to explore new ideas, beliefs and cultures. Rebellion is the name of the game; just make sure your actions are for a purpose, and not just for the sake of being rebellious. This is a great moon to shift old stuck patterns and look to a new way of being. This is a time to encourage new thoughts and ideas to flow through your projects or magical practices.

MOON IN PISCES - THE FISH

* *Mode*: mutable Water sign
* *Key phrase*: "I receive"
* *Ruled by*: Jupiter
* *Body parts*: feet and lymphatic system
* *Gifts*: sensitivity, compassion, imagination, intuition
* *For the flying ointment*: work with mugwort and fly agaric on a Piscean moon

When the moon is in Pisces, there is a really romantic, soft atmosphere, as though our boundaries and edges are blurred. This can be an emotionally sensitive moon, and retreat and quiet may be necessary. This is a time to be kind and considerate to yourself and draw in softness and ease through magic.

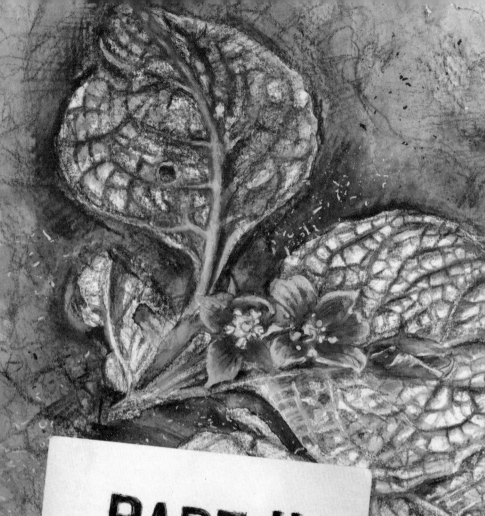

PART II
CONNECTING TO THE WITCHING HERBS

"ALL HUMAN BEINGS HAVE MAGIC IN THEM. THE SECRET IS TO KNOW HOW TO USE THIS MAGIC..."

SYBIL LEEK, WITCH, ASTROLOGER AND PSYCHIC (1917-1982)

Getting acquainted with plants is one of the most powerful acts of magic you can perform. You begin to enter their world and walk down the path of intuitive communication with them. In this part of the book, we will be outlining some of the ways in which you can deepen your relationship with the power plants. We will also be getting to know the witching herbs themselves, focusing in particular on henbane, datura and belladonna – their subtle energies, biological make-up, their histories and mythologies and the various ways we can work with them medically and magically. As hexes have a long association with the witching herbs, we will conclude this part of the book with a very specific hex that is aimed ultimately for the good of all.

- 4 -
THE MAGIC OF PLANT CONNECTIONS

o you talk to plants? Interactions arise when our senses respond to the plant's chemical compounds, and a delicate dance of communication begins. Our physical body may react to their phytochemical compounds; for example, a herb may be soothing for the throat because of its mucilaginous compounds or stimulating for the digestion if bitter in taste. They can also profoundly affect our mental states.

There are subtle energetic responses at work. Plant magic can be sensed, felt and experienced but not explained with words or measured in a linear way. Every living thing emanates an electromagnetic frequency determined by its chemical make-up, the environment – and some inexplicable magic.

We can sense when life is in flow, bliss is in bloom and synchronicities occur, just as we can sense feelings of being stilted. Working with plant magic can give us a framework to shift stuck patterns and create healing in our lives. It can facilitate a reconnection, a time for reflection, letting go and moving on.

Whether you enjoy placing your hands in the soil, your pencil on paper or your mouth to the pipe, there are never-ending ways to connect with plants. You can never get bored and the journey never ends. We will be introducing ways to connect with plants, which we encourage you to use in your work with them.

MAGIC OF PLACE

Native and traditional practices the world over have been influenced by the landscapes, plants and habits of the people who live in them. If we are to live harmoniously within a landscape, interacting with its plants is essential for our survival. With this in mind, as we come to understand the workings of our green friends and the ways in which they grow, we can develop rituals that are reflective of the messages of the environment that cradles us. Within the space in which we walk, there is a resonance with the rituals that have been carried out there from time immemorial.

To work with the witching herbs requires knowledge, experience, courage and trust. They can also be considered channels to the witches of the past, as they invite you into their magical and mysterious realms. There is increased potency when you learn to frame your magical work and rituals with whatever nature and the Universe gifts you. Likewise, the influence of celestial bodies of our solar system on life and the world around us are part of our landscape, above and of the Earth.

The ethereal kiss of enchantment is most delicious when we create the time, space and connection to check in with ourselves, our quest and environment, thereby deepening self-awareness and self-care. There are different rites and rituals we can carry out to focus our attention on one intention, to enhance our clarity of thought and to help to engage the Universe in our needs and desires. Making use of tools and specific herbs means that we can explore altering our state of awareness or consciousness to connect with the power of nature and spirit all the more readily through rituals. However, our connection with the landscape and the secrets it holds can start with something as simple as the cultivation of the plants themselves.

MAGIC OF CULTIVATION

Growing and planting out herbs is a sacred form of creativity. We Seed Sistas learned this early on as children – especially from one grandmother in particular who was a keen and brilliant plants-woman, and who talked incessantly to each and every one of her beloved plants, calling them her babies. We relish sweet memories of the supreme care taken over worms in the soil; the need to talk to the trees and bushes, shrubs and seedlings; the careful formation and mixology of the compost heap; the attention to detail in the literal shit, the muck and manure that fertilizes our food and medicine;

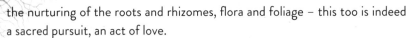

the nurturing of the roots and rhizomes, flora and foliage – this too is indeed a sacred pursuit, an act of love.

Sensory Herbal Magic encourages the growing of plants; in fact cultivation is an essential aspect of the whole process of understanding plants. When you create an opening for the witching herbs in your life, inviting them into your gardens and psyche, the plants are perceptive and respond, appearing as if out of nowhere. A spell can be cast with each and every seed germinated, an intention to draw peace and health to our planet.

You too can be shown so many secrets and stories by the witching herbs simply by collecting their seeds, and bringing them home to germinate and grow in your grounds, plots or surrounding wild lands. Then comes the wonderment of watching the first leaves appear, the growth of the plants, sitting with them, listening to the murmurings of the tales they tell through their rich and ancient folklore, weaving new narratives into the fabric of our lives. Plants can even appear and connect with you in your dreams.

The ability of plants to respond to their environment has a scientific name: gnosophysiology. Plants sense their environment and react through adjusting their form or shape (morphology), their internal processes (physiology) and their characteristic or expression of the changes (the phenotype). They are able to learn from, and adapt to, the world around them.

Plants react to a range of stimuli such as humidity, temperature, pathogens, gas concentrations of carbon dioxide and oxygen, insects, physical injury and light, to name a few. Plants also respond to humans; to voice, sound, breath and emotion expressed through changes in the electromagnetic pulse emanating from the heart. This is why talking and singing to our plants is so vital – and opening our voices to be conduits for cosmic forces yields surprising delights. We have had a fair few eureka moments when letting words stream through us.

PLANTING THE FIRST SEED

When looking up witching herbs such as henbane and belladonna in books, you will find that they are often categorized as "poisons" and labelled "toxic". As a result, many people shy away from digging any deeper and discovering their lessons. There is stigma associated with these power plants, so lifting the veil is vital; as is opening new dialogue with all plant lovers about these much-maligned beauties. Some people are concerned about having poisonous plants in the garden where children play. To this, we say: educate children to recognize the plants; bring them into the garden and help them build a rapport with these beautiful souls. One of the most stunning woodland and cottage-garden plants in Britain is the foxglove. Children are usually warned to keep away from this attractive beauty but it certainly isn't banished from gardens countrywide.

It may be trickier to teach your pets to recognize the witching herbs, but the potato and tomato plants belong to the same family of nightshades and their leaves are toxic to pets. Keep an eye on your furry friends and if you suspect they have ingested any of your plants, take them to the vet. The witching herbs generally have a bitter taste (owing to the alkaloids), so hopefully animals are unlikely to eat enough to cause any lasting issues. Signs that they've ingested these plants include drinking lots and drooling, followed by lethargy.

Growing these plants is the best place to begin opening new paths of understanding. The gathering of seeds, germinating them, planting, nurturing, harvesting them, and processing the medicine – each individual task can be a sacred ceremony, attuning our attention and focus so we are fully present.

The cycle of a plant's life begins with the seed, which will germinate and pop out a baby rootlet, the radicle, to start anchoring it to the ground. The seed's leaves emerge, with the first distinct pair of leaves bringing additional energy for the growth process. Roots establish, leaves grow, flowers emerge to be pollinated and will then turn to fruit and seed, ready to start the cycle again, over and over. In Sensory Herbalism, we follow and observe the plants through the seasons and the autumn or fall represents the seed time for us here in Britain, packed with the power for potential, inspirations and ideas.

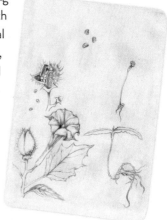

SEED PLANTING RITUAL

A seed is a physical representation of pure magic. From this dormant, fertilized plant ovum, new life will sprout, creating the potential for many more generations (or variants) of the parent plant to spring forth.

Steps:

1. If you have not already harvested your henbane, datura and belladonna seeds (usually prepared in early spring), you can source them from select plant nurseries.

2. Prepare your seed by energetically potentiating the little miracle on your altar. You can voice your wishes for its new life; maybe there is specific magic you wish to do with the plant as it grows or things you will create from the plant as it develops, which you can focus on now.

3. Further prepare yourself for planting by having a ritualistic smoke (see page 76 for more information).

4. Read and educate yourself about the most auspicious time for planting. There are various theories you can explore such as biodynamics, which is a holistic, ecological and ethical approach that takes notice of the astrological phases. This attention to detail will aid your new growth projects and connect you to the land and your seed.

5. When you have chosen the best time for planting your treasure, begin the process of germination by soaking the seeds in water (which will help to soften the hard coats of some seeds and leach out any chemical inhibitors that may prevent germination) and leave them out in the moonlight one night before planting.

6. Place the soaked seed in your mouth for a few minutes while you focus on thoughts of the plant growing powerful and healing medicine.

7. Infused with your own DNA, the seed can finally be planted in the Earth, where you can closely observe it grow into a plant. When choosing how and where to plant it, you will need to consider certain factors:

   *   Where is the best place for this plant to grow – in shade or sunshine?
   *   If you are planting your seed in a garden, in which direction is it facing?
   *   Will you start your seedlings off in pots? Or put them straight into the ground?
   *   What is the best type of soil for this plant – sandy, moist?
   *   How will you protect your plants from frost or slugs, or other potential threats?
   *   Do you have a watering system?

There is more on the specific cultivation of three of the Solanaceae plants in their dedicated chapters, and instructions in Chapter 13 on harvesting and drying herbs for magical use.

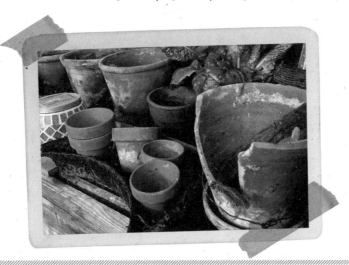

OPENING THE GATEWAY – RITUALISTIC SMOKE

Planting and harvesting rituals have been a historic part of societies dependent on good crops and harvests for survival. The ritual preparation of seeds and growing practices are wonderful ways to begin a connection with some of the more powerful and poisonous plants, especially since you will not always ingest these herbs. It is not essential to imbibe a plant to learn about its medicine.

There are many ways to mark the opening of a ritual. We choose the ancient global practice of producing sacred smoke to initiate, potentiate and bless our work. We always draw on our trusted friend mugwort and love working with her in a smoking rite before planting seeds and harvesting the herbs. While mugwort is our herb of choice for burning or smoking, there are many others, one of the most famous of all being henbane, which we will explore later.

SACRED SMOKE DOWN THE AGES

Ritualistic smoking has been documented in many ancient cultures and evidence has been found in ancient burial chambers. This was from long before the arrival of tobacco from Virginia to Europe. Traditionally Indigenous Americans smoke tobacco in the ceremonial "Peace Pipe". This is a ritual process that historically has taken place when talks were being held between tribes to settle disputes. Tobacco is considered a sacred and powerful plant.

The tribal users of tobacco, among the people from where it originates, have an understanding of the tobacco spirit. Tobacco use wasn't intended for habitual use; rather tobacco was invited for specific sacred situations and to build a connection between people. This is a far cry from the state of affairs created in our modern world of consumer capitalism and vast addiction to smoking commercial cigarettes or inhaling chemical vapes. At the time of writing there is an important movement throughout the Nation Native Networks to keep tobacco sacred.

Among the Indigenous Americans of the plains, Peace Pipes are contained in a bag called a pipe bundle. This bundle was decorated on the outside and was used to carry the tobacco that would be smoked in the pipe. *Chanunpa*

is the Sioux name for the sacred ceremonial pipe and the ceremony in which it is used.

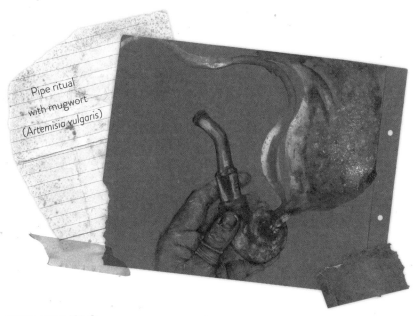

Pipe ritual with mugwort (Artemisia vulgaris)

PIPE RITUALS

In the Western magical tradition, a pipe ceremony is a sacred ritual for connecting the physical and spiritual worlds, and can be both satisfying and magical. The fire in the pipe represents the sun – the source of life. The bowl of the pipe represents the receptive principle, open to inspiration; the shaft, the directive energy of intention. The pipe links the heavens to the Earth, letting our intentions for the harvesting of the medicine become physical.

The smoke creates an atmosphere and, depending on what is smoked, can alter your state of consciousness. The smoke becomes your intention; it wafts out, touches everything and carries prayers into the ether. The whole pipe and the act of smoking symbolizes a union and a balance between being open to receive and yet having clear intent. Like us, you might choose to have a pipe ritual before your work with plants to focus your intentions.

Over the years, we've experimented with many plants that can be smoked. Some that are high in resins, such as calendula, can induce headaches and not feel good for the body. Then there are many other herbs that smoke smoothly, delighting the senses. While some herbs may alter consciousness, there are many that are free from the addictive compound nicotine.

You may be concerned about the health implications of inhaling herbs. With any heat going into the throat rather than vaporizing, there is the potential for cell transformation that can lead to mutations in the throat mucosa – but this occurs with regular daily use and we are not suggesting mugwort pipes as a replacement for tobacco addiction or the daily smoking of herbs, as there are specific times for connecting with divinity and attaining the desired effects.

There is no legal age for smoking herbs although many places selling herbal tobaccos will act with discretion and not sell them to under-16s. Enjoy and celebrate the pipe ritual with care and intention.

It is very difficult to regulate the dose when smoking the three powerful witching herbs, so this is not recommended for use in medicine.

MUGWORT, A MAGICAL FRIEND

Many moons before the nicotine plant arrived in Europe, people smoked mugwort. Mugwort is popularly known as gypsy's or sailor's tobacco. The plant's Latin name, *Artemisia vulgaris*, is based on that of the Greek goddess Artemis, a powerful ally indeed. Artemis is a moon goddess, ruling over the night skies and connecting us to the dream state. It's interesting to note that mugwort has been linked with pineal-gland stimulation and gently alters the state of perception too. Ancient cultures smoked mugwort to promote vivid dreams and it can produce a mild psychotropic effect while awake. Smoking mugwort is an age-old practice and can connect us with our ancestors.

The Divine Nature of Mugwort

We have seen how mugwort is connected to the goddess Artemis. Mythological connections and associations like this can help to open up our understanding of the power plants.

Interestingly, the Egyptian counterpart to Artemis is Bast or Bastet, who was originally depicted as a lion-headed woman and believed to protect against diseases. She was particularly caring toward women and children, vanquishing all threats from malevolent spirits. Like Artemis, she held the nature of duality in her soul and as time ticked on she became depicted as a domesticated cat, but she is still at heart as fiercely protective as a lioness.

Smoking dried mugwort in a pipe can help you to gently open up, receive nature's gifts fully and communicate on a slightly different level. When working with herbs for medicine and ritual work, it is important to be in an open, receptive state to be able to communicate with the plants. Mugwort aids this sense of openness. When you light the mugwort pipe, gentle plumes enliven the senses and mark the start of the work.

Mugwort
(Artemisia vulgaris)

Smoking mugwort is a timeless and beautiful practice that can deepen our connections to the herbs. Mugwort does not contain nicotine, is non-addictive and its tar levels are considerably less than those of tobacco. Many choose to use smoke without inhaling, which can still create some of the desired outcomes when performed with smoke bundles or incense. You can draw on mugwort in various ways: burning dried bundles or a charcoal disc as part of an incense blend.

CLEANSING SMOKE AND INCENSE

Smoking has always been a part of ritual, whether it's done with a pipe or by burning rod bundles or resin on a charcoal disc. Bringing herbs and resins together with fire and creating fragrant protective smoke opens and holds our magical practices.

The long tradition of using smoke to clear out unwanted insects and mites is an ancient one and is also applied as a spiritual practice to get rid of unwanted energies. Herbal smoke can be employed to create a sense of cleansing in the environment and of your own energy fields. When, for example, we've seen a challenging case in the consultation room, utilizing herb smoke is an effective way of creating a clear and cleansed atmosphere. There has been more recent research to show that through this process, ions alter in the air to create a negative charge, the same change that is created when a flock of birds takes off. The air becomes less dense and reactive.

The use of smudge sticks for creating cleansing smoke has become a popular practice in modern Western spiritual practice. Smudge sticks are generally made from white sage and their use stems from Native American tradition. The recent surge in the use of the term "smudging" has come from a Western interest in Native American practices and has often been diluted, while sources of white sage become endangered as demand has increased. Masses of "smudge sticks" are sent worldwide from the USA, and little is fed back to profit the original communities. There is current interest in protecting white sage stocks as well as a call for recognition of the origins of these practices, to ensure that Indigenous communities can properly benefit from such widespread use.

We don't have to appropriate the traditions of other cultures to benefit from the effects of practices such as the use of ritual smoke. In the UK and Europe, there is a long tradition of burning herbs for protection and reaching altered states, but it has been forgotten down the centuries, and perhaps even occluded by modern interpretations of "exotic" practices from far-off lands. The Gaelic word *saining* means to use a charm or smoke for blessing, protecting or consecrating a space, while *reeking* is an Anglo-Saxon word for creating smoke. The Old English word *rec* originally meant "smoke from burning material", and it wasn't until the 17th century that the word "reek" acquired the sense of stench. We Sistas have named our mugwort smoke bundles "Reeking Rods", and we sometimes burn these bundles in place of smoking a pipe as part of our ritual preparations.

Depending on what it is you burn, different emotional and psychological effects can be created in the person who inhales the smoke or enters the room afterwards. Think of the effect of frankincense used in churches, for example, or sandalwood in a Hindu temple. The word "incense" describes smoke with a scent and comes from the Latin word *incendere*, meaning "to burn". Generally, the word has become synonymous with resins such as myrrh, sandalwood or frankincense. Resins were burned by the ancient Egyptians seemingly for both practical and more esoteric reasons. The antimicrobial and insect-repellent properties of resins support health where sanitation is more challenging, while the inhalation of resin smoke can alter the state of consciousness, which is why resins were often burned during religious rituals.

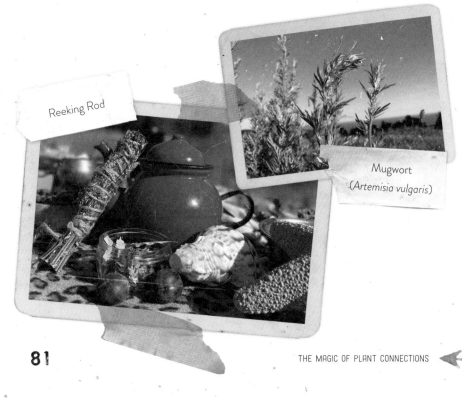

Reeking Rod

Mugwort
(*Artemisia vulgaris*)

HARVESTING AND DRYING MUGWORT FOR SMOKING

Mugwort is at peak power during the summer months. The best time to harvest the flowering tops is at the time of an Aquarian full moon in August, on a dry day after any dew has evaporated.

If you wish to make your own mugwort tobacco, the first thing you need is a positive identification of the herb. Mugwort can be confused with a few others in the family such as wormwood or tarragon, so spend some time learning the botanical features.

Steps:

1. Take scissors or a knife and cut the herb in lengths of about 70cm (30in) to 100cm (40in). As you harvest it, you may like to hum or sing and enter a meditative space to connect with the plant, letting mugwort know this harvest is to become your sacred smoke. You can commune with the plant and be open to discover what exchange may be applicable. We often ask, "What is it that I can do for you?"
2. Tie your fragrant bounty into bunches and leave it to hang in a well-aerated space away from direct sunlight or intense heat.
3. After a week to 10 days the herb should be dry enough to strip from the stems. This is a ritual in itself, so lay out a large sheet, put on some music and work gently and consciously, stripping the leaves and blooms away from the stems and branches. Observe how the herb looks and how this whole process feels.
4. When you have obtained your leaves and blooms, work this plant material with your fingers into smaller and smaller particles – again you can sing your prayers into this.
5. Store the mugwort in dark glass jars or tobacco tins, label with the name of the plant, the date and any intentions you may wish to bring to your sacred smoke.

Awareness Around Spiritual Practices

When people first tap into the spiritual world, connect with others, open up to nature, maybe take mind-altering plants and fungi, they can become like sponges, absorbing practices, terminology and beliefs shared by people they admire. It is our belief that practices and terminology should be checked for authenticity, ecology and impact on the planet, and to understand where items come from and with what intention. For example, the word "shaman" has its roots in Siberia, yet has become a blanket term for many variations of psycho-spiritual practices that may have little or no relation to these origins.

In the modern world, cross-pollination of cultures, ceremonial ideas and artefacts is inevitable. In Sensory Herbalism, we have been influenced by many medicine traditions around the world. We are constantly learning ourselves and aim to practise discernment when it comes to understanding what we are partaking in and perpetuating in the world; we are focused on decolonizing our own minds as much as possible and are open to learning where we have been brainwashed. We suggest that if you feel too uncomfortable to ask questions about the origins of knowledge, preparations and practices, or if the answers you are given are not satisfactory to you, seek out people, plants and places that feel more honest and open. We can choose to self-govern in these areas to ensure that we are part of a gentle and transitional movement aiming to decolonize ourselves.

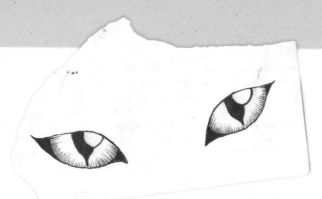

STORYTELLING WITH PLANTS

Through observing plants as they grow, their habitats and how they manifest physically, we can connect with the life force of each plant's character, spirit and entity, and create deep relationships with our floral friends. Plants are like people, each with their very own personality traits. Some you like, some you don't; some you fall in love with and some you fear. By recognizing these emotions, you can begin to draw parallels with friends and family members and start to see how certain types of people resemble certain types of plants.

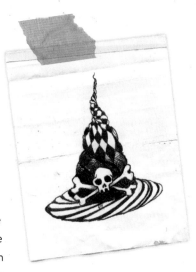

The more time you spend deeply observing and working with the power plants, the deeper your friendship develops, the more familiar their character becomes and the more their medicine reveals itself to you. As your witching herbs grow, you may want to sit with your new buddies and talk to them.

After personal relationships with the power plants have been forged by planting and growing them, we recommend that you discover the folklore around them, which contains both wonderment and warnings in a way that can be understood on a visceral level. Their stories hold great power and can be used as therapeutic tools. These narratives carry the experiences of medicine and magical people through time and hold the key to the remedies and energies held within them. Working in this way is a personal healing experience in itself.

The stories associated with each of the witching herbs contain layers of knowledge, teaching us science, magic, nomenclature and sensory understanding. The passing on of sacred knowledge is one reason that stories develop around the plants, as this helps to carry their messages and magic down through the generations. Stories are reinvented with each repetition and naturally morph in order to stay relevant to each new generation; but as long as the storyteller is also working with those plants, the essence and meaning of the stories won't get lost. There is a beautiful synergy when we engage our capacity for creativity and storytelling to animate the lessons that plants can teach us and the medicine they impart. Applying concepts or words to the narrative enables better memory recollection.

Telling stories about the plants is a way of spreading your knowledge in a fun way, for a storyteller is much more than a teller of tales. Storytellers are important entertainers, teachers and healers. As one of humanity's oldest art forms, storytelling both stimulates the imagination and builds a strong sense of kinship between all present at the telling of a tale.

We can find stories everywhere – in the news, our books, on television and the internet. Everyday conversation is full of anecdotes and real-life stories. Storytelling helps us contextualize and comprehend our environment and personal experiences on a more visceral level.

Stories can be mysterious and mighty. Many older stories are originally traditional folktales. They represent the richness of oral patterns of telling and are the product of a community experience, as well as the art of the individual storyteller.

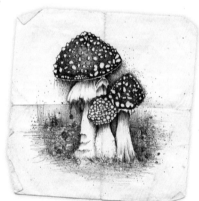

Historical tales, legends and contemporary works can be the subject of the storyteller's tale, and they too embody a strong element of community or collective experience. They contain hidden messages to support and guide communities, sometimes even to control them.

The emphasis of traditional storytelling is as much on the act of telling as the story itself. True storytelling happens when it is told person to person, live, without print or technology. Nothing beats the experience of a live performance when bringing tales to life. The story does its magical work in silence. What stories do you know that contain plants? Do you know the one about the twelve swans and weaving nettle shirts? Or the one about the magic porridge pot?

In Chapters 6 to 8, we will be sharing some of the stories that have helped us to understand the characters of these wonderful plants, and we would encourage you to create your own stories too.

THE NAMING OF PLANTS

There are many stories to be found on the naming of plants. The Swedish botanist Carl Linnaeus (1707–1778) was responsible for the development of the binomial nomenclature system of Latin plant names in the 18th century that we still use today. Within the Linnaean system, a plant's first name is written with a capital letter and denotes the plant's genus, such as *Rosa*. The second name is its species and is written in lowercase, for example *canina*. The plant's whole Latin name is then written in italics, as in *Rosa canina* – more commonly known as the dog rose. The system includes plant families, which are not given in italic. In *Rosa*'s case, this would be Rosaceae or the rose family. Linnaeus then extended his system to the animal world too, such as the name for humans – *Homo sapiens*.

Binominal nomenclature is a hotly debated topic that may well have been deconstructed and reworked over time. Linnaeus lived at a time of peak colonialism and there are plenty of questionable ideas within his approach, for it was also the era of pre-Darwin theories on evolution. He led the way to scientifically classify humans into different races or species according to their place of origin and skin colour, placing white Europeans at the perceived top of the pile. He was part of the long history of patriarchal white supremacy that relates to all botanists and so-called "plant hunters" of the Linnaean era. While the system still stands and he is integral to its history, it is important to recognize the atrocities of the times.

Linnaeus's model was considered remarkably modern for the age. Bridging religious and scientific concepts of nature, he set about ordering the world in what he considered to be the clearest way. At the time, Latin was seen as a language that could be recognized the world over. Today, while the folk names of plants still differ from region to region, the Latin name and species remain the same. Thus the system provides a language for discussing plants across nations or between counties where they may have different common names. It is vital that local names of plants are recorded and continue to be used. Each one of the common names holds stories and clues to their medicinal uses.

As we saw in the case of mugwort, a number of the botanical names of our plants derive from Greek and Roman myths, and from the stories of gods. So even in a scientific system, the stories break through. The flower aster, for example, is named for the star goddess Aster, who looked down at the Earth from her heavenly place and was saddened when she saw it had no stars of its own. She wept over the Earth, and where her tears fell, the asters bloomed.

THE LANGUAGE OF FLOWERS

From the time of the ancient Greeks onward, people have created stories and characterizations about plants and attributed symbolic meanings to them. It is said that the language of flowers originated in Middle Eastern harems where the written word was forbidden and secret messages were transmitted through the giving of bunches of blooms.

In the 19th century, there was great interest in creating tales about the plants. Over 150 floral dictionaries were published during the period in Britain, ascribing thousands of flowers to a particular vibe or energy. This meant that when a lover or a friend brought you a bouquet, there were underlying messages contained in the colourful, scented gift. While a red chrysanthemum could mean "I love you", a daisy signalled innocence and a sheaf of corn would foretell the promise of riches, some of the powerful poisonous plants brought a different set of meanings. The following examples are from Kate Greenaway's *The Language of Flowers*, published in 1884:

* a gift of mandrake signified "horror"
* foxglove brought a promise of "insincerity"
* henbane shouted "imperfection"
* belladonna signified "silence"
* datura symbolized "deceitful charms"
* wolfsbane linked to "misanthropy"
* hemlock meant "you will be the death of me!"

Wolfsbane
(*Aconitum napellus*)

WEAVE YOUR OWN TALE

You will find that each of the witching herbs is very much alive and willing to interact with you, especially as you grow and nurture them, inviting them into your heart. You will notice their individual traits, how they differ from one another and what similarities they share. You may find that you wish to contribute to their folklore by weaving your own tales about them.

Steps:

1. Let yourself daydream about what sort of person/ animal/deity/entity the plant is.
2. You might create your own names for them. Belladonna might get shortened to the nickname of Bella or Donna or Dark Lady or Fate – whatever you personally connect with. Or maybe there is a completely different name that rings true with the character traits you assign to the plant.
3. What kind of friends, lovers or children do they have? What kind of life have they led?
4. What might their story be?
5. Could you write it down and share this story with others?

If you would like to read an example or two of these sorts of stories, you will find characterizations of our three nightshades in Chapters 6, 7 and 8.

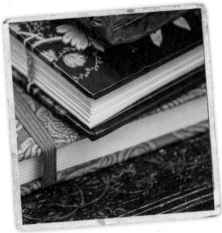

Anthropomorphizing and Genderization in Storytelling

Attributing human characteristics to plants is another topic of much debate and discussion. We Seed Sistas use characterization to connect with the plants and their spirits. This often includes genderization – ascribing gender to objects and cosmic forces. (Depending on your "mother" tongue, you may already do this.) We sense gender when working with herbs; this has to do with the social conditioning of our upbringings, the associated folklore around the herbs and our experiences growing up as women.

Nature is interpreted through the eyes of your current paradigms and the modern stories of the plants can reflect that. Our intention is to give life to new lines of nature story that are relevant to the paradigms we live in. On our courses, people have ascribed different gender expressions, or seen their plant characters as genderless sprites, beings or energetic expressions of the plants. Now we are learning about non-binary terminology as the world shifts to catch up with less rigid binary gender expressions.

Some argue that genderizing the plants can feed into patriarchal impressions of female and male characteristics, limited by a language that assigns one set of characteristics to the masculine and another to the feminine. Yet calling plants "it" can feel disconnected, so the American author and botanist Robin Wall Kimmerer has suggested a new pronoun, "ki" (meaning he/she/it), and plural, "kin" (for they/them).

Botanically speaking, most plants are hermaphrodite (can reproduce from a single plant), even if some of them – hazel, for example – keep their different functioning flowers (the male and female flowers) apart. Some plants are dioecious, meaning they have either male or female flowers, but not both. If the pollen is transferred to the "female" plant, fertilization occurs. For example, female holly plants produce berries when they are fertilized by pollen from a male plant. The common nettle is another example of this, hence the plant's Latin binomial name, *Urtica dioica*. *Dioica* translates as "two houses", referring to the male and female plants.

In your own storytelling, let yourself be guided by what the plants reveal to you about themselves.

HERBAL OBSERVATIONAL DRAWING

A large part of Sensory Herbalism is based around uniting and bonding your own energy with that of the plants by creating observational drawings of them. Time and time again we witness wonderful art from everyone, each an expression of creativity unique and incredible. Every individual is gifted profound learning through their artistic observations. Especially when it comes to the power plants, drawing them offers possibilities of deepening a relationship when it isn't safe to imbibe them regularly compared to other less potent plants.

When becoming still to observe a plant – form, colour and even its subtle movements – we discover new knowledge. If you draw a plant in detail you will never mistake that plant for another when you are out on a walk. You will see the plant on a subtle and insightful level, thus beginning the process of truly meeting the plant. You notice the tiny hairs that may be present, the shapes present in the leaf veins like the tiny repeating hearts in comfrey leaves, or the eye-like iris patterns in the centre of dock roots ...

It is through drawing the plant parts that we first noticed henbane's five-petalled flowers have mesmerizing dark veins that swirl with patterns reminiscent of our own microvasculature. The sticky hairs on the leaves have no uniformity of length and have parallels with old men's untrimmed nasal hairs! If you are drawing henbane's multiple seed heads, you will witness for yourself the similarity to our own jaw bones and teeth. There is much humour in the henbane and you might find yourself laughing out loud as you sit and draw.

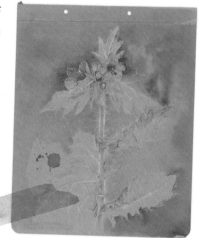

DRAWING PLANTS

*For this exercise make sure that you give yourself time – take
a moment to turn off your phone and be fully present.*

Steps:

1. If you find the plant out in the wild and can comfortably sit nearby,
   then do so. If you are drawing a potted plant, place the pot in
   the centre of a table or somewhere you can look at it closely.
2. Observe the whole plant and draw its silhouette or outline.
3. Observe how the plant is growing. Do the branches reach upward?
   How might the environment have affected how the plant grows?
4. Sit with the plant a little longer and you might sense the plant's
   energy. Is the energy condensed and shimmery, or flowing and wispy?
5. Choose a particular aspect of the plant to focus on. For example, you
   could draw one of the leaves, taking note of the veins and margins.
6. As you draw, take notes of things that pop up in your mind.
7. After drawing the plant write down the botanical name
   and common names and perhaps the date or season.

Alongside your drawings, and provided there is
enough leaves or flowers for you to take a couple
without harming the plant, you may wish to stick
a dried leaf, flower or some seeds into your art
book for future reference. To dry them out,
simply press the plant material between two
sheets of printer paper or kitchen roll and
then place this between two sheets of baking
parchment. Put the sheets in the centre of
a heavy book and leave for a week or two.

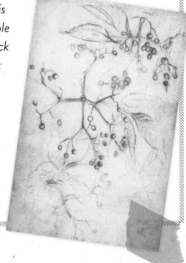

MAKE YOUR OWN FLOWER PRESS

If you have the right tools you can make your own flower press ...

You will need:

* 2 A4-size boards of plywood or MDF
* a screw gun or drill with drill bits the same diameter as that of the wing nut bolts
* a pencil
* 4 wing nut bolts approx. 12cm (5in) long
* wood glue
* 5 sheets of thick card
* scissors
* 10 or more sheets of double-ply kitchen roll or printer paper

Steps:

1. Drill a hole in each corner of your first board. The holes should be just wide enough for a bolt to fit through and around 1cm (½in) from the edge of the board.
2. Place the first, drilled board on top of the second. Use a drill bit or a pencil to mark through the four holes to show where the holes need to be on the second sheet in order to line up. This second lot of holes should be slightly wider than the bolt diameter. Take note of which way round you have the boards to ensure they continue to line up.
3. Drill the four holes in the second board, which is going to form the top cover of your press.
4. Removing the wing nuts, push the four bolts up through the holes in the corners of the first board, which is going to be the bottom cover of the press. You can glue the bolt heads in place on its underside.

5. You have now created the outer covers of the press, which you can decorate if you wish.
6. Next, trim the sheets of thick card and cut off their corners so that the sheets fit within the central area created by the four bolts coming up through the bottom board.
7. Now place your first sheet of trimmed card on the bottom board. Follow this with two sheets of paper and then another layer of card, two more sheets of paper, another piece of card and so on, until you get to the last piece of card.
8. Place the top board on top of the paper and card by shooting the bolt shafts through the drilled holes and use the wing nuts to secure firmly in place.

Your flower press is now ready to use. When you wish to press flowers, remove the top board and place your flowers or leaves between the sheets in the press. Then replace the board and tighten the wing nuts once more.

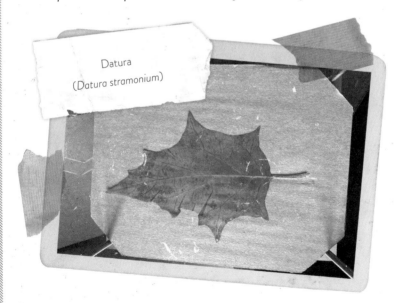

Datura

(Datura stramonium)

CREATE YOUR OWN MANDALA

Using a sheet of paper or card, and several different types of plant and plant parts, e.g. roots, seeds, leaves, stems and blooms, you can make a form of meditative art called a mandala. "Mandala" is a Sanskrit word that originally meant a circular figure symbolizing the Universe in Buddhism and Hinduism. Today, it can refer to an abstract design that often comprises a series of concentric circles linked by geometric patterns.

You can turn plant parts into a potent mandala symbol of your own. Start in the centre of your image by laying out and gluing seeds in a circular pattern on your paper or card. Then move out from there, using leaves, flowers, stems and roots, before using seeds again. Take your time and reflect on what you are doing.

Mandalas can look stunning and are a great way to connect creatively and meditate on plants and their life cycles.

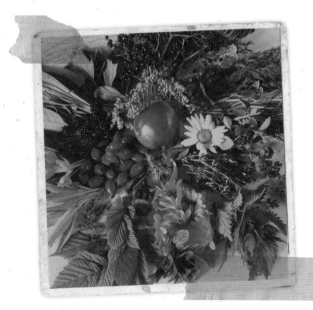

A POWER PLANT GRIMOIRE

Why not create your own beautiful witching herbs grimoire
filled with your observations, illustrations, poetry (your
own and other people's), incantations and notes?

Steps:

1. If you wish, invest in, or make your own, flower press and preserve
    these glorious beauties so that you can add them to your book.
2. Make a plant mandala picture to display on
    your altar or include in your grimoire.

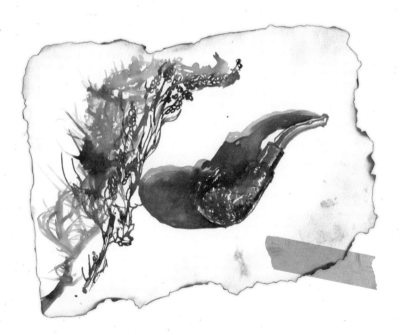

CONNECTING WITH PLANTS THROUGH SPELLCRAFT

Spellcraft can beautifully and creatively add power to magical work. In an ideal world we would flow through life bending away from challenges, like water flowing round obstacles, but sometimes the cumulation of life's difficulties can cause a feeling of walking through mud, surrounded by a thick fog, and the way through is hard to visualise. If you are suffering from stuck feelings, need some luck or help with love, travel or work, all these can be aided with a good spell. The care and energy taken in this craft creates an awesome atmosphere which helps us to feel even more connected with the subtle energies and aligned with the vital forces. Consider how you are interacting with nature and what you are offering back, as this brings more potent energy to the work. Reciprocity is key. We must support love and give back to nature as we ask for the universe for clarity and support.

Spellcraft defines and makes our intention and spiritual forces visible. It can be any ritualistic act that we do with attention and intention, taken to invoke a response within our lives.

You can bring spellcraft into your ritual work with the power plants – from the collection of their seeds through to planting, tending, harvesting and creating potent potions. Ritual and devotion moves through all of the work. Spells don't have to be complex or involve expensive tools; the practice is linked to the attention taken, what is offered and the setting of clear intentions.

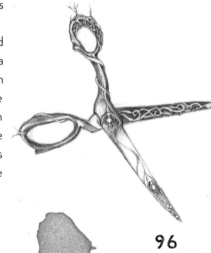

The spirits, cosmic forces and associated deities of henbane, datura and belladonna support certain energies that we can summon for our spells, as we will see. Invite powerful deities to bring forth certain shifts in your life with full awareness. These energies hold intension through the ages and you are tapping into a mighty force. Be sure you offer your respect in exchange.

CONNECTIVITY AND COMMUNICATION
WITH COSMIC FORCES SPELL

This spell is best performed when the moon is transiting either Gemini or Virgo, the mercurial signs of communication.

Steps:

1. Choose one or more dried mercurial herbs (e.g. valerian, fennel, marjoram, dill or lavender) to work with.
2. Cast your circle for protection.
3. Write your name next to the feeling of flow and connectivity. Start to draw a figure of "8" around each of these labels, joining them together.
4. Trace with your pen or walk this live around the opposing forces until they seem to merge through the path you are drawing. Sprinkle your herb over the "8" with your name in one side and the sense of flow and connectivity in the other!

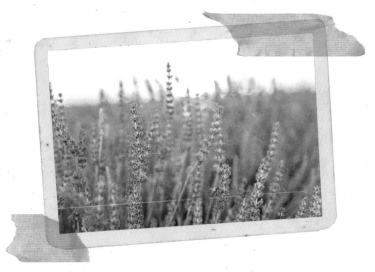

- 5 -
THE COMPLEX NATURE OF
THE WITCHING HERBS

 s we have discovered, the witching herbs have developed a fearsome reputation for being shady magical mediators as well as potent medicinal agents. As with all herbs, their medicine elicits a physical reaction and the plants of the nightshade family that we have been looking at – henbane, datura and belladonna – can all be applied in clinical herbalism to exert medicinal actions on tissue that is in spasm.

However, there are also the more emotional and spiritual actions that can be elicited from them too. Our work with these plants over the years has led us to our own conclusions; while there are established physical indications or patterns of response for the herbs we are looking at, each one has its own individual energetic picture. Thus these plants can be prescribed to create subtle changes in the energetic field interacting with neural pathways to cause specific responses. They can be applied for specific emotional and spiritual healing.

In this chapter, we will look at their biological make-up and their subtle energies. We will see why they are linked to poison, yet have potential for healing.

THE NIGHTSHADE FAMILY

The Solanaceae plant family, or nightshades, consists of over 2,500 different species and are found on almost every continent of the globe and in almost every habitat – from rainforest to deserts.

For all that nightshades are known as plants of ill-repute, it is important to put this oft-feared plant family in perspective. You might not realize that you eat plants daily that share characteristics with some of the most powerful poisonous plants. The vast nightshade family consists of tomatoes, aubergines, peppers and the humble potato – common fodder on millions of platters worldwide. Also included are chilli and coffee, stimulating the masses. The truth is that important members of this vast plant family feed and energize our global population.

POSSIBLE ROOTS OF THE FAMILY NAME

Although they have the collective name of "nightshades", not all of the Solanaceae plants flower by the shade of night. The origins of the Latin plant family name, Solanaceae, are unclear, but might stem from the Latin word *sol*, meaning "sun", possibly referring to the certain members of the family's sun-resembling flowers. Another possibility is that the root was *solare*, meaning "to soothe" (or *solamen*, "a comfort"), which would refer to the slumber-inducing effects of the plant upon ingestion, and also their pain-relieving qualities.

NIGHTSHADES AND ALKALOIDS

Nightshades contain chemical compounds known as alkaloids. The word "alkaloid" itself comes from the term "vegetable alkali", referring to the alkaline nature of these compounds. (Remember those science lessons at school, and studying pH values, where alkaline sits at the other end of the spectrum from acidic?) The alkaloids are a diverse group of medically significant compounds, which include well-known drugs such as opiates (sourced from the opium poppy).

Isolated alkaloids generally have a strong bitter taste, which means that they tend to act as digestive stimulants in humans, yet have also been shown to protect plants from destruction by certain insect species. Alkaloids have the ability to cross the blood–brain barrier, thus creating powerful effects on consciousness and emotion. They generally have a marked action on humans or other animals.

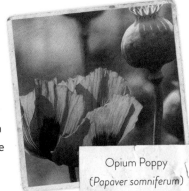

Opium Poppy
(*Papaver somniferum*)

WHY PLANTS HAVE ALKALOIDS

It has generally been assumed that alkaloids are a by-product of plants' metabolic processes. It has now been shown that a concentration of alkaloids in some plant species increases dramatically just before seed formation and that these appear to participate in their metabolic processes. Let's go back to the humble yet mighty potato. They turn green, increasing in alkaloid content, just before sprouting.

Of course, the potato is a member of the nightshade family, and the Solanaceae as a whole are characterized by their high content of potent alkaloids, which is connected to both their healing power and their potential toxicity. All the nightshades are therefore potentially toxic, depending on the dose in which they are administered. Remember the poisonous nature of the green skin of sprouting potatoes? Also consider the powerful stimulating nature of coffee beans, the relaxing nature of tobacco or the endorphin-releasing properties of the chilli ... Even the most seemingly innocuous members of the family can be seen to exert powerful effects on the human body.

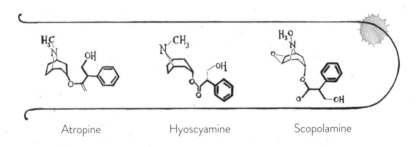

Atropine   Hyoscyamine   Scopolamine

ALKALOIDS AND THE NIGHTSHADES

Okay, so this next bit is pretty geeky. We've tried to provide a simplified breakdown of why the body responds in the way that it does physically to certain plants in the nightshade family. The more magical and emotional responses to the herbs can never be fully understood or broken down in this way, but if we can understand how the plants work physiologically on the nerves in the body, we will have a more holistic understanding of them – and perspectives from many different angles.

Plants in the nightshade or Solanaceae family contain a specific class of alkaloids called tropane alkaloids. These compounds provide much of the altered states of consciousness and the physical medicine of the witching herbs. Studying them can help us to understand the physical responses experienced when ingested.

The tropane alkaloids, scopolamine, atropine and hyoscyamine, are found in varying amounts in different genus of the Solanaceae.

All three of the Solanaceae herbs we are looking at in this book – henbane, datura and belladonna – contain tropane alkaloids in varying amounts. Alkaloids are a type of active compound found in plants. Tropane comes from the Greek *tropos*, meaning "taking a turn'" or "adopting a new manner". This indicates the transformative nature of these compounds.

The tropane alkaloids are fat-soluble, which means they are easily absorbed through the skin. In humans, tropane alkaloids interfere with the functions of the chief neurotransmitter Acetylcholine (ACh), which is the most common neurotransmitter. Broken down, neurotransmitter means neuro – nerve – and transmitter. It's like a tiny chemical messenger in the nervous system making sure one nerve talks to another and tells it what needs to happen!

THE WITCHING PLANTS AND THE CENTRAL NERVOUS SYSTEM

In the central nervous system, the neurotransmitter ACh acts as part of the cholinergic system in the brain. It is one particular pathway of nerves that serves a specific function. Our view of the world around us is in part shaped through how we respond to ACh, as it is associated with a number of cognitive functions: attention and arousal, learning, memory, selective attention and emotional processing. ACh is therefore allied with conscious awareness (that is, our understanding of who we are and our place in the world). Pretty amazing! That tiny chemical compound enables nerve pathways to link together so that we know (or think we know) who we are and what place we have in the world.

When we interfere with this cholinergic pathway, we interrupt these cognitive functions. During tropane alkaloid intoxication – such as that caused by large doses of our beloved Solanaceae plants – we can become cut off from some of the links to certain cognitive functions. This could be seen as revealing deeper aspects of the brain and allowing us to function more directly from the limbic and reptilian brains. We can, in effect, start to reveal our more animalistic, emotion-led, ancestral parts of ourselves that we were yet to become aware of.

BALANCING OUR BASIC INSTINCTS

We humans might think ourselves sophisticated, but our responses to our environments are often involuntary and the majority of our bodily responses take place without conscious effort and oftentimes without our awareness. Our autonomic nervous system (from the word "autonomous", meaning self-governing) affects our heart rate, digestion, respiratory rate, salivation, perspiration, urination and sexual arousal. It's also responsible for the "fight, flight or fright" response, and it largely acts independently of our control.

When the fight, flight or fright response is initiated by the autonomic nervous system, noradrenalin and adrenalin trigger a series of responses in what gets called the sympathetic nervous system. In however small or large a way that the response is activated, the neurotransmitter ACh is produced, which then initiates the opposing response. This is called the parasympathetic response and is an attempt by the body to maintain homoeostasis or balance.

In this opposing response to re-address balance, ACh performs a wide range of actions, from initiating the constriction of the pupils to decreasing heart rate, like a natural pace-maker. When these pathways are interfered with, for example by the tropane alkaloids (in the Solanaceae), the following actions can occur in varying degrees:

* pupil dilation
* decreased saliva production
* decreased mucous production

* increased heart rate
* relaxed bronchial muscle
* reduction in gastric juice secretion
* decreased urine secretion but relaxation of the bladder wall and tightening of the bladder sphincter
* decreased digestive secretions and motility in the digestive system

This means that the body and mind may respond in seemingly contradictory ways to the tropane alkaloids. For example, at higher doses, someone could be lying down and appear relaxed with limp muscles, but their heart could be racing and they could be hallucinating.

THE ALCHEMY OF HENBANE, DATURA AND BELLADONNA

Back to our tropane alkaloid-containing herbs, henbane, datura and belladonna, which all contain varying amounts of the tropane alkaloids scopolamine, atropine and hyoscyamine. Each alkaloid has been found to act in slightly different ways on the body, having an affinity with different organs due to their receptor sites. As a result, depending on the relative amounts of alkaloids in each herb, they in turn affect different areas or even specific organs within the body. The wisdoms passed down the linage of British herbalists is that datura has a specific affinity for the lungs, henbane for the mid abdomen or the peripheries and belladonna for the lower abdomen.

Datura
(*Datura stramonium*)

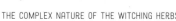

Asthma Cigarettes

Medicinally, one of datura's more famed uses is for the respiratory system, specifically as a bronchodilator. In 1802, British physician and asthmatic James Anderson visited India, where he enjoyed a mild relief in his breathing after smoking a cigarette containing *Datura stramonium*.

Anderson returned to England and reported his find to his friend Dr Sims in Edinburgh. Sims trialled the remedy, noted the benefits and published a report in the *Edinburgh Medical and Surgical Journal*. As a result asthma cigarettes entered into the British and American pharmacopoeia, and became popular for the treatment of asthma.

The herbal company Potters started to make asthma cigarettes with lobelia, datura, belladonna and henbane that could be bought at any chemist without prescription.

In the 1970s and 80s, with the rise of the punk movement and increased exploration of psychedelics, thanks to Carlos Castaneda's publications, countless numbers of people experimented with Potters asthma cigarettes. As people were unsure of dosages and without guidance, there were unfortunately many hospital reports and anecdotes of these easily bought and accessible asthma cigarettes causing Solanaceae-induced mania and anticholinergic syndrome (see page 109).

EFFECTS AND USES OF THE COMPOUNDS

There is, of course, much cross-over with the actions of henbane, datura and belladonna because of the compounds that they contain. When you smell the leaves of these herbs, there can be no mistaking the fetid alkaloids they have in common – albeit in different quantities.

The levels of these also vary throughout the plants' growing phases. In *Datura stramonium* (a species commonly found in the UK), it has been suggested that young plants contain principally hyoscine, whereas hyoscyamine is the principal alkaloid at the time of flowering and thereafter. In belladonna, it appears that hyoscyamine is the dominant alkaloid throughout the plant's life cycle.

The relative amounts of these alkaloids can also vary with climate, daylight hours and chemical sprays. We must keep in our minds that these are isolated compounds and not the whole herbs themselves. Herbs contain many compounds that work synergistically in the whole plant.

Each of the individual alkaloids atropine, hyoscyamine and scoplomine acts in different ways and for different amounts of time.

HALF-LIFE OF THE TROPANE ALKALOIDS:

The term "half-life" is used to measure the length of time it takes for half of a drug to be excreted from the body, so a longer half-life means more long-lasting effects.

* Atropine – 2.5 hours
* Hyoscyamine – 3.5 hours
* Scoplomine – 8 hours

EFFECTS AND USES OF ATROPINE

* Used therapeutically to reduce activity in the Gastrointestinal (GI) tract
* Blocks cholinergic innervation to sweat glands
* Reduces hypermobility to the bladder
* Used to decrease salivation and dilate the pupils
* Produces varying effects on the cardiovascular system

EFFECTS AND USES OF HYOSCYAMINE

* More potent than atropine in its peripheral and central effects
* Used as an adjunct in the management of peptic ulcers
* Reduces gastric secretions

THE COMPLEX NATURE OF THE WITCHING HERBS

EFFECTS AND USES OF SCOPOLAMINE

* Acts as a central nervous system (CNS) depressant at therapeutic doses
* Prevents motion sickness
* Blocks short-term memory and can be used during anaesthetic procedures
* Therapeutic indications include GI anti-spasmodic, anti-emetic, anti-arrhythmic
* Adverse effects: blurred vision, dry mouth, flushed appearance, anxiety, irritability, insomnia

PHARMACEUTICAL MEDICINE AND THE COMPOUNDS

Due to their strong effects, the tropane alkaloids have been used in pharmaceutical medicine to treat a wide range of conditions – ranging from Parkinson's disease to heart conditions. Interestingly, they are even used to treat the side effects from anti-psychotic drugs and as an antidote for the overdose of cholinergic drugs or mushroom poisoning.

As with any medical intervention, there can be side effects, from glaucoma to memory problems if the alkaloid penetrates the central nervous system (especially in the elderly). Every medicine needs to be handled with respect and care – and those offered by the nightshade family are no exception.

BREAKING DOWN CONDITIONING

These three Solanaceae plants can help us to peel away our conditioning and interpretations of the world that occur as a direct result of us existing in society. Their chemical compounds can disrupt some of the pathways of acquired knowledge and return us to deeper, more hidden aspects of ourselves.

However, in cases where people are looking for a recreational experience of altered consciousness, the Solanaceae are notoriously difficult to use; the risk of a physically detrimental overdose is high, and the effects are unpredictable. These plants can connect with our intuitive self but also the murky parts of our psyche and ancestry that lay hidden deep within. Solanaceae intoxication has

Henbane
(Hyoscyamus niger)

Belladonna
(Atropa belladonna)

Datura
(Datura stramonium)

often resulted in visions of people covered in hair and is thought to be the root of the werewolf myth. The hallucinations can be deeply unpleasant or confusing, and visual hallucinations can continue for several days after consumption.

On the other hand, when respected and used in small doses these plants can be applied to access these very same fears and help us to recognize and integrate them as they arise. Diving into the depths of our psyche can bring awareness of the fears we have and where they stem from.

It is no coincidence that henbane, datura and belladonna thrive in barren landscapes and inhospitable soil. All three are the possible culprit when people are paralysed by neurosis and fear renders it almost impossible for life to flourish. And all three offer differing insights in how to move through our paranoias and fears by releasing the emotions and exposing a more primal instinctive self; trusting in the unknown, embracing the mystery.

DOSAGE OF THE WITCHING HERBS

In our herbal practice, we recommend using sensory drop doses. We want to connect people to sensory experiences with herbs rather than encourage the use of large, pushy doses of herbs, which can be too forceful or aggressive.

Clinically and recreationally, we have always worked with small drop doses to encourage subtle neurological shifts. In a single sensory dose there are few actual compounds ingested; however, they are extremely effective at triggering immunological or energetic shifts. The dose generally doesn't contain enough compound to be poisonous, or to interact with pharmaceutical medication.

Anything that is sensed by the body can evoke a response via our internal systems. The autonomic nervous system and endocrine system adapt our internal environment to the external environment. They pick up cues from our senses to prompt such changes. And so the compounds from medicinal plants send diverse cues and we react in diverse ways.

Small doses act more energetically than large ones; they stimulate innate physiological, neurological and hormonal responses, and affect the subtle energy patterns of the body, mind and spirit. As the dosage increases, the effects of the herb become more gross, more rooted in the material.

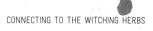

UNQUENCHABLE THIRST

Anticholinergic syndrome occurs when the dose of the herb or alkaloid is too high. We Sistas have experimented with much higher doses on ourselves in the name of research, and soon learned about the effects of anticholinergic syndrome. It results from the inhibition of cholinergic neurotransmission (see page 110). Usually the first sign of anticholinergic syndrome is an unquenchable thirst. This would be an indication to cease use of the alkaloid or herb until symptoms abate.

If, however, the anticholinergic syndrome is initiated, there are some symptoms to expect, including dilated pupils. There was a ditty developed to aid the diagnosis of anticholinergic syndrome in the hospital setting. It goes like this:

"Blind as a bat,
(mydriasis or pupil dilation)

Mad as a hatter,
(delirium)

Red as a beet,
(flushed skin)

Hot as Hades,
(fever)

Dry as a bone,
(dry mouth, dry eyes and decreased sweating)

Heart runs alone,
(tachycardia, i.e. rapid heart rate)

Bowel and bladder lose their tone."
(losing control of excretory functions)

THE COMPLEX NATURE OF THE WITCHING HERBS

WHAT TO DO IN A POISONING

If the Solanaceae are consumed in excessive doses and poisoning does occur, symptoms will be very uncomfortable and may include dry mouth, headache, light sensitivities, hallucinations, bladder retention, fast heartbeat, vomiting, dilated pupils, difficulty swallowing, hot dry skin, unquenchable thirst, dizziness, tremors, fatigue and problems with coordination. As we have seen from the half-lives of the alkaloids, specifically scopolamine, anticholinergic syndrome can be long-lasting. In these instances, seek professional medical advice immediately.

Once medical attention has been sought, the Rosaceae family, which is high in tannin content, can be drawn upon to speed up recovery. Alkaloids are precipitated out of a liquid by tannins, which cause them to chelate. This makes them almost totally non-absorbable. In accordance with this mechanistic idea, this would mean that any herbal mix containing herbs with high levels of tannins (for example, the Rosaceae family) would render the alkaloids inaccessible to the body. Tannins can also, therefore, serve as a useful immediate treatment for acute alkaloid overdose.

Prevention is better than cure. Keep poisons (whether in the form of tinctures or other preparations of these plants) away from children and people who may swallow them accidentally.

If you are growing these herbs in your garden, educate your children and all people who pass through about what they are and explain why it is not a good idea to ingest these plants.

In any type of poisoning, there are some basic steps to follow to offer support and clear toxins from the body, described below.

POISON MANAGEMENT

Dosage for poisoning can vary greatly according to a person's size, situation, how much or what they've eaten that day and how sensitive they are to the toxin. In the event of poisoning it is important to seek professional help as soon as possible. If you are with someone that has overdosed on the Solanaceae, they may be feeling extremely frightened or out of control. Try to calm them down with a sweetened tea while outside professional help is sought.

Here is a checklist and a few techniques to help manage poisoning cases.

* Stop any causative agents, such as ingesting a toxic tea, for example.
* Take their pulse rate – it will be increased in anticholinergic syndrome.
* Pay attention to the maintenance of their airway, breathing
  and circulation, and call an ambulance immediately if
  there is any sign of a dangerous physical response.
* Reassurance and management in a quiet area may be
  sufficient for those with mild signs/symptoms.
* Phone your national poisoning helpline.

When dealing with poisonings, there are a range of techniques that can support the body's systems to eliminate harmful compounds and keep the nervous system calm. If you are working with any plants regularly, we recommend having a first-aid box to support a multitude of situations. If treating poisoning, consider what resources you have to hand, the length of time since ingestion and what additional tools or skills you have that might be relevant in the situation. Here are some steps that may help recovery in mild cases:

* Giving regular sips of green clay in water will help to
  chelate (i.e. make them bind to it) and expel alkaloids,
  reducing the amount entering the bloodstream.
* Expelling the contents of the stomach is recommended
  but this can be challenging in the home situation.
* Make a green vegetable juice containing lots of celery
  to support the kidneys and increase excretion.
* Reflexology points can help to relax and eliminate,
  massaging over the points that relate to the liver,
  intestines and the kidney areas in particular.
* Herb bathing rituals such as adding a pot of a yarrow infusion to
  the bath can help to eliminate toxins and encourage circulation.

A CLOSER LOOK AT ODYSSEUS'S MOLI

We mentioned earlier the mythical tale of Odysseus, who countered datura poisoning with a remedy called "moli", which has links with the snowdrop. The snowdrop belongs to the Amaryllis family, whose compounds have been researched as a potential treatment for Alzheimer's disease. Some of the symptoms of the anticholinergic syndrome caused by the Solanaceae alkaloids can be likened to certain types of dementia.

The Odyssey may be a fictional story, yet it expresses some knowledge of the plant medicine that existed at the time it was written. It could be that Odysseus's counteracting of the effects of datura occurred from the vomiting induced by the snowdrop, but it is more likely that there are interactions between the two plants at the level of the neurotransmitters. Where datura has anticholinergic effects, snowdrop has compounds indicated for their cholinergic effects, which are useful in the treatment of Alzheimer's. Datura blocks ACh on receptor sites, while snowdrop increases levels of ACh by preventing its breakdown. This could be an important indicator for members of the Amaryllis family in acute tropane alkaloid poisoning, but there are obvious toxic implications with the snowdrop indicated by vomit induction on ingestion. This definitely warrants further investigation.

PHARMACEUTICAL ATROPINE POISONING

After pure atropine alkaloid was first isolated in 1833, poisoning inevitably occurred – whether deliberate or accidental. The largest collection of clinical cases ever compiled was by the American physician and toxicologist Rudolph August Witthaus in 1911. He described a series of 682 individual cases, 379 of which were caused by preparations of belladonna (in the guise of eye drops, plasters or liniments) and 303 by the pure alkaloid atropine. More than 500 of these poisonings were deemed to be accidental. There were also 37 suicides and 14 murders connected to atropine poisoning. The number of total reported deaths was 60 (approximately 12 per cent). This was before the days of intensive care and mechanical ventilation. Since 1911, and Witthaus's classic series, atropine poisoning has become rare.

Susceptibility to the toxic effects of atropine varies widely. Death can occur after as little as 100 micrograms, yet instances have been described where the patient has survived after taking as much as 500 micrograms. Children are more sensitive to the alkaloid and infant death has occurred after as little as 10 micrograms by mouth.

THE MAGICAL THREE

With their similarities and their differences, henbane, datura and belladonna are triplets whose very individual characters complement each other in many ways. The number three itself represents a portal, a gateway, into another realm – from one the singular, to two the partnership, to three taking us into the many. Three is playful; you can create patterns with three. The number three has always represented the spirit of magic and long been considered lucky.

Throughout human history, the number three has always had a unique significance. When we think of time we have a past, a present and a future; thus stories including our own often fall into three parts. Folklore, mythology and fairy tales with roots that tap deep into the psyche so often comprise the number three: three bears, three billy goats, three wishes from the genie, three-faced goddesses, three kings, and so it goes on ...

The number three has roots in the meaning of multiplicity. Creative power; growth. Three is a moving forward of energy, overcoming duality, expression, manifestation and synthesis. Three is birth, life and death. Three is a complete cycle unto itself of past, present and future.

For the Greek philosopher Pythagoras, three represented completion. It is composed of the beginning (1) and the middle (2), which add together to create the end (3). The number three is the only number equal to the sum of its previous numbers and thus signifies prudence, wisdom, piety, friendship, peace and harmony. The triangle represents balance and is a polygon of stability and strength.

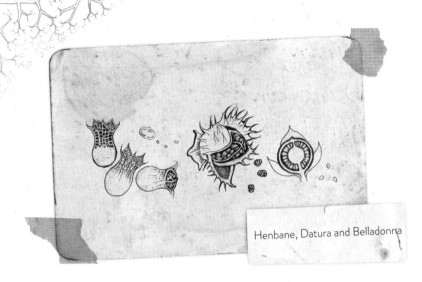

Henbane, Datura and Belladonna

THE TRIPLE WITCH POISONS

In our journey with henbane, datura and belladonna we will be sewing together threads that tell a story, with the intention of reintegrating these powerful medicines into clinical and traditional herbal practice today.

These three-tropane-alkaloid herbs all have valuable physical actions as well as the ability to induce altered states. In one aspect, they interact with cholinergic pathways to elicit certain physical and psychological responses; while from another perspective, these herbs offer us an ethereal ability to step back in history and tap into the archaic practices of our ancestors.

In the chapters that follow, we will get to know our three more closely. We will learn more about how henbane has been used for anaesthesia, numbing pain and relieving fears. It can also be used to aid in embracing one's own death, bringing joy and celebration where there was once fear and anxiety.

We have touched upon how datura has been used to treat asthma and tremors, but we will also see how we can use it for understanding different aspects of the self, for delving deep, for introspective work.

Belladonna has long been associated with causing death and poisoning, with eye surgery, curses and cures. We will discover how its beauty can connect with endings and finality – allowing a new cycle to begin.

Dramatic Poisonings

William Shakespeare suggests that the poison put in the ear of Hamlet's father was henbane. In Act 1, scene 5, the ghost of Hamlet's father explains:

Thy uncle stole

With juice of cursed hebenon in a vial,

And in the porches of mine ears did pour

The leperous distilment; whose effect

Holds such an enmity with blood of man ...

Shakespeare also describes belladonna's poisonous qualities, in particular the plant's ability to cause a coma-like trance. In the final act of *Romeo and Juliet*, our tragic heroine takes a potion to fake her own death and place her into a catatonic state.

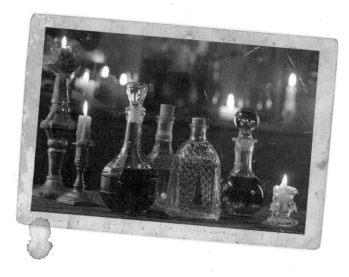

THE COMPLEX NATURE OF THE WITCHING HERBS

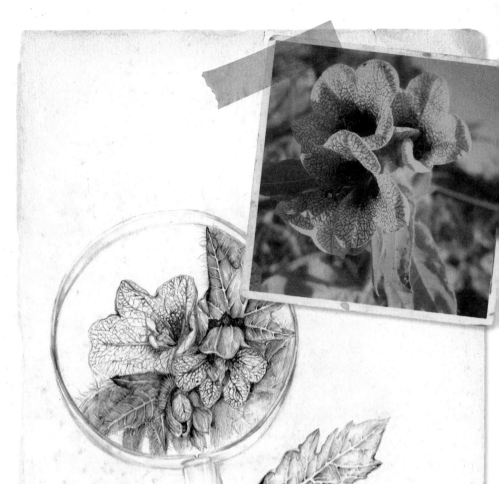

HENBANE

HYOSCYAMUS NIGER

– 6 –
HENBANE
MESMERIC BEAUTY

ne of the most famous medicines and esteemed magical plants, Henbane was familiar to ancient authors the world over. This mesmeric and intricate floral beauty is, in our experience, the most uplifting and jovial of the three Solanaceae plants we will be shining the spotlight on in the following three chapters. Associated with "celebration of death", henbane has the power to bring a sense of joy and playfulness where there was previously bottomless despair.

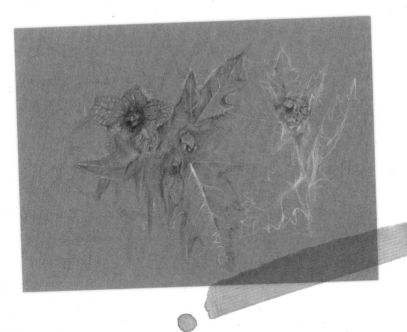

Latin name

Hyoscyamus niger

Common names

Black henbane, Jupiter's bean,
hog's bean, stinking nightshade,
herbe aux dents (from the French
for "toothed grass"), devil's eye

Astrological ruler

Jupiter

Actions

Anodyne, anti-anxiety,
anticholinergic, antispasmodic,
aphrodisiac, diuretic (mild),
narcotic, sedative, soporific

Etymology

The genus name *Hyoscyamus* derives from the Greek *hyoskyamos*,
meaning hog bean; in some parts, hog's bean is still a common name
for *Hyoscyamus niger* today. The herb was ascribed to the super
strong Hercules who has been depicted wearing a crown of the plant,
representing his ability to travel to the underworld.

The botanist Linnaeus gave henbane the name *Hyoscyamus* in 1753.
He based it on the former more illustrious name of *dioskyamos*,
meaning god's bean.

Henbane's Germanic names of Bilsner and Bilsenkraut come from
links to Norse mythology, specifically to the goddess Bil. Stories tell of
her ability to bridge worlds in colours of light. In the early Germanic
language, bil may have meant "vision, hallucination" or "magical power,
miraculous ability"; a nod to the potential of henbane as a powerful
mind-altering plant.

Distribution

There are many different species of henbane around the world. In
this chapter, we will focus on *Hyoscyamus nigra* (back henbane)
as this is the species that we most commonly cultivate.

GETTING TO KNOW HENBANE

Our valuable medicinal ally is often described as an evil-looking, stinking malodorous weed. The cheek of it! This dark description gives henbane a sinister reputation, as indeed is the case with all the witching herbs. Around the time of the Middle Ages, even just having these plants in your garden could be enough to get you brought in for questioning about sorcery and witchcraft. Much had changed since the times of the ancient Celts and Greeks, who considered henbane sacred to the upbeat powerful sun gods Belenus and Apollo respectively, and a herb that walked in the light. It was during the times of the Inquisition that a Christian wave of suppression induced fear and loathing of the very plants that had been synonymous with healing, personal empowerment and beneficial medicine. The time has come for us to strip away the mask of fear that covers henbane, and truly honour this friend in a more open-minded and sensitive way.

Henbane has been revered by many different cultures and ascribed to diverse gods – from the dark Hekate to the luminous sun deities. The famous oracles at Delphi were said to inhale henbane incense in order to divine the future in a state of ecstasy. In the more northern European lands, the Druids and bards inhaled the smoke to travel to the realms of the Fae and otherworldly beings.

In Sensory Herbalism we highlight how people can build their own relationships with plants using their full senses, intuition and close observation, working closely with the plant material and only imbibing super-small dosages. Without fail, when people connect with henbane in our group settings, it initiates feelings of lightness, chatting and laughter, and there is a willingness to talk about reactions to this plant in a jovial, animated way, in comparison to the more introspective attitude brought out by datura, for example. Here follows a character profile created with the storytelling technique described in Chapter 4.

MEET HIERALDO HENBANE

Hieraldo Henbane is a completely timeless and ageless gentleman, with the best sense of style; a super-dapper individual, dressed in pale linens and silks, always fresh. His voice is that of a hypnotist, so tuneful and melodic that it has the power to lull you into deep relaxation.

Hieraldo is highly intellectual, well read and accomplished. He has been a trained anaesthetist since youth, going on to practise both dentistry and surgery. He has gifts of seership and many people make a pilgrimage of sorts to his home for insights. As they sit around the large oak table with his trademark incense burning, he brings forth the deepest mysteries from each participant's life, uncovering truths and futures previously untold.

Hieraldo's parties are legendary and everyone clamours for an invite, knowing the beverages on offer hold dreamlike delights. His home is opulent, on the banks of the wide and mysterious River Styx. Some revellers never return from festivities at his infamous house.

He has a fiery temper and when he gets irritated he must be appeased; otherwise things seem to combust around him. He has a wild wanderlust.

KEY THEMES FOR HENBANE

The word associated with henbane in Sensory Herbalism is "wake"; the celebration of death of a life past. In this celebration, delight and pleasure can be found even in the darkest places. Henbane is not for heavy introspection but more for moving away from pain, welcoming joy and seeing the light that can guide us through times of shadow and shade.

* For relieving pain and fears – of death in particular
* Embracing own death
* Bringing joy where there is dread and anxiety
* Jovial spirit
* Relaxing spasm
* Opening up
* Connection with the dead

THE HISTORY OF HENBANE

Henbane has been written about widely in historical texts for a range of applications including helping us to sleep, read the future, lucid dreaming, incite passions and of course to talk to the dead.

An early Anglo-Saxon record refers to the sedative properties of henbane, stating, "If a man cannot sleep, take the seed of henbane and the juice of garden-mint, mix together and smear the head with it, he will soon be better."

During times of the witch persecutions, the majority of which took place in the 16th and 17th centuries, henbane was often used in evidence that the wise women were telling fortunes and dispensing aphrodisiacs. (Sounds like our kinda people!) A henbane decoction aided the wise women most often deemed witches to invite prophetic dreams and divine futures.

Oleum henbane, an age-old aphrodisiac massage oil made from the leaves of the plant, incites lust. The lust-enhancing oil was famous in the folklore of the witches of Thessaly, a region of ancient Greece. In addition to its aphrodisiac intent, the oil contains warming and pain-relieving properties. We Sistas still make this archaic preparation today and can attest to both the pain relief and the incitement of desire!

People didn't have bathrooms at home in the Middle Ages, so there were public facilities that, according to reports, were very fruity places. In Italy, they were frequented by prostitutes called bordellos and were centres for good, "clean" erotic fun, excuse the pun! In them, henbane seeds were strewn over glowing coals to heat up the erotic atmosphere. The smoke, mixed with steam, appears to have induced strong aphrodisiac effects. (Makes throwing a little eucalyptus essential oil on the sauna coals seem positively boring ...)

After all the washing some deemed it necessary to get dirty once more and dig up a dead body or three. Necromancy has historically been practised by peoples to commune with their dead loved ones, as ghosts were believed to hover in the vicinity of its corpse's place of burial. Henbane has been written about in literature pertaining to necromancers, who used it to invoke demons and the souls of the dead. To commune with the deceased, handfuls of dried henbane plant material and seeds were thrown on hot coals, producing a sacred smoke to open up lines of connection. Necromancy is still explored by some today and a few still draw on henbane to enhance this practice of magic and communicate with the deceased – either by summoning their spirits as apparitions, or conjuring visions to discover their hidden knowledge.

Besides using henbane for magical purposes, the herb had everyday uses, such as in brewing – the results of which can, admittedly, still have transformational powers ...

BREWING WITH HENBANE

Alkaloid-containing plants such as henbane were used by ancient cultures to strengthen beer. We take it for granted these days that beer and ale are made and flavoured with hops. But until the general adoption of hops, beer was made with a wide variety of herbs, and the fermentation and the brewing of beer has long been linked with psychotropic herbs. For example, the ancient Egyptians brewed with mandrake, dried fly agaric was added to beer in Siberia, thorn apples in Russia, opium in China and henbane was used in Europe.

Henbane brews can introduce a sense of the extraordinary into daily life, and induce vivid illusions in a waking state. After drinking henbane beer, very real yet mundane hallucinations can occur. One night, after we drank henbane beer, we spent many hours looking for a cat that we don't own – a cat that didn't exist. We did, however, get a cat unexpectedly a couple of months later, so could the experience have been some sort of a premonition? Even if you are used to lucid dreaming, henbane beer, as is often the way with the Solanaceae, will take away any awareness that you are dreaming.

Henbane was used in the form of a traditional herbal gruit (a herb concoction used to flavour beers, usually bitter) before the first ever drug law of the Beer Purity Act was introduced in Europe in the early 1500s, which decreed that only hops could be added to beer. With the rise of Puritanism and the Protestant Church came a movement to stop brewing with the traditional herbs of the times. We do not know exactly for how long humans had been brewing with henbane prior to that, but possibly for over 5,000 years. At an early brewery site in Skara Brae, Scotland, archaeologists found residue of a beer made with henbane and meadowsweet. Before the Beer Purity Act, there had been large demand for the henbane herb in Germany and northern Europe specifically for the production of beer; thus specially designed and managed henbane gardens sprang up all over the place and were considered holy. Microbreweries were plentiful; in fact most households potentially brewed their own intoxicating henbane tipple.

Medieval mystic, abbess, herbalist and botanist Hildegard of Bingen wrote in the 12th century that hops "make the soul of man sad, and weigh down his inner organs". When you compare hops with henbane, it is clear that after the Beer Purity Act a much more sedative and numbing herb was added to beer in place of an uplifting and psychotropic plant. Hops caused the drinker to become drowsy, and diminished sexual desire. Imagine the shift in energy this change produced in community celebrations, festivals and rituals.

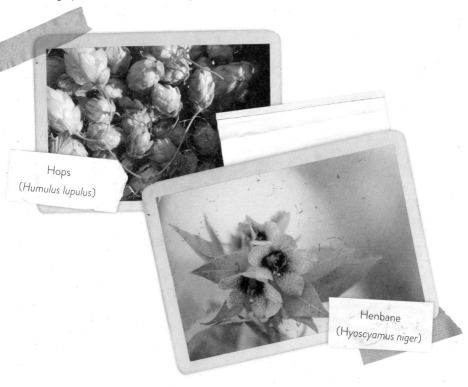

Hops
(Humulus lupulus)

Henbane
(Hyoscyamus niger)

UNCLE VICTOR'S HENBANE BEER

Victor is a dear friend of ours – an alchemist brewer who creates charmed beers and ales deep in the Dorset hills. He shared the following recipe with us and explained how brewing beer can be either a simple exercise or an extremely precise process. Making henbane beer is probably as old as the craft of brewing itself and, as we've seen, was once extremely common. In our experience henbane beer has a very strong and bitter taste. However, the brief and basic version of the brewing process shared here is for information purposes only – to give you an idea of the process, rather than to use as a recipe.

Steps:

1. Mix barley with water heated to 150°F/65°C in a mash tun (a pot used to make a porridge). This converts the starches in the grain into sugars that can then ferment.
2. Leave for an hour then sparge (wash hot liquor/water through the barley) to collect as many of the sugars in it to ferment into alcohol.
3. Put in a copper pot, adding hops and any other herbs, and boil for an hour or two. This is now considered the "wort" – a solution of extract made from grain to be used for fermentation by yeast into beer.
4. Crash-cool the wort after the boil and put in the fermentation tank where yeast is added and fermentation commences.
5. Remove some of the wort and add dried henbane in what's known as "dry hopping". This is added back to the main batch before fermenting further.
6. The fermentation process takes place over a few days and then the beer will be allowed to mature to make it smoother.

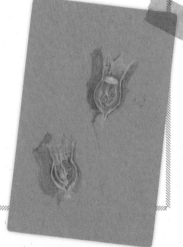

HENBANE'S MYTHOLOGY – SEX, WAR AND DEATH

As will be clear by now, henbane is a rock-and-roll plant associated with carnal lusts and extravagant, ritualized orgies, or communing with the dead in darkened graveyards. Henbane deals out heightened awareness and pleasure. However, the plant may also lead us to war, and there is hot debate among academics as to whether or not henbane was used by the Vikings on their rampages.

It has been argued that the much feared, indomitable warriors known as the Viking Berserkers may have drunk potions made from henbane and/or other nightshades to induce their wild and violent states when going into battle. There has been much supposition about what could have led to the Berserkers' ruddy faces, wild abandon and ability to deal with pain, all of which fit the henbane intoxication picture. They were said to have taken henbane before battle as a "herb of courage". They were feared for being merciless, killing all in their path, seemingly unaffected by injury to themselves.

In some Chinese texts, henbane or *Làngdàng* is infamous as a hallucinogen, while the seeds are referred to as heavenly transcendent. To reduce the toxicity of these seeds they were prepared for medicine by soaking them in a milk and vinegar preparation. According to the classic Chinese medicine text the *Shennong Bencaojing* of 200 CE:

> The seeds when taken, properly prepared, for a prolonged period enable one to walk for long distances, benefiting to the mind and adding to the strength ... and to communicate with spirits and seeing Devils. When taken in excess, it causes one to stagger madly.

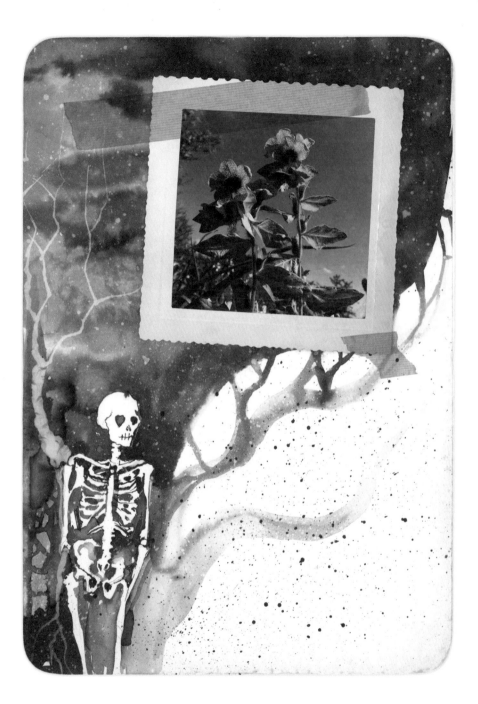

Henbane Cultivation

Henbane is one of the most mesmerizing beauties of the Solanaceae world. The flowers are generally creamy in colour with deep purple veins running throughout the five petals. There is not a person who can look at the flowers in bloom and not gasp at the intricate patterning on the petals. The stem is hairy with large alternate leaves that are irregularly lobed. The root is a tap root. The whole plant has that amazing Solanaceae scent that becomes so familiar when you grow them. The plants range in height from 2–4 ft (60cm to over 1m).

Interestingly, the henbane plant can be either annual or biennial. To make matters more confusing, both types of plants result from seeds from either annuals or biennials. There is a theory that the annual plants result from seeds from the first flowers while the biennial plants result from seeds from flowers produced later in the summer. We have never been able to successfully try out this theory and we have mainly grown annuals.

Henbane enjoys the margins, the edges of fields, often enjoying this broad view of the world. The plant does not need rich soil but rather seems to prefer poorer-quality soil. It will happily share a pot with another more nutrient-dependent species, as happened once when henbane self-seeded in with an avocado tree we kept outside our front door.

If you wish to cultivate henbane in your own plot or garden, for successful growth it requires a poor-quality and well-drained soil and an open, sunny space, but it does not want much attention beyond keeping the ground free from weeds. In fact, they love to be neglected and often self-seed on waste ground.

The seeds are numerous and light brown in colour with a reddish tint. They are as tiny, or perhaps slightly tinier, than the poppy seeds many of us are familiar with from cooking. These minuscule seeds packed with potential are said to remain viable for over 600 years. Pharmacological experiments have shown that the seeds of the henbane are super potent! Not only do the minuscule dots possess all the medicinal properties of the entire plant but have ten times the strength of the leaves because the alkaloids (see Chapter 5) become condensed within them.

These seeds can be scattered on the surface of the soil, but you can sow them in a pot if you wish (see the practice below). In the northern hemisphere, they can be sown outdoors in early May or as soon as the ground is warm.

To sow indoors, place the seeds in the fridge for a couple of weeks before you plant them to emulate the colder night temperatures they would experience outdoors. This is called stratifying the seeds. Before planting, you can soak the seeds for a few hours to deactivate the enzyme inhibitors and thereby allow the seeds to germinate.

HARVESTING HENBANE

The exact time to harvest will depend on the maturity of your plant's growth, but we prefer to harvest when the plant is in flower. You don't want to miss out on seeing the flowers of henbane, for they are a sight to behold, and resemble the pattern of veins beneath the surface of an elder's thin skin. The phase of the dark or new moon is the best time for harvesting leaves from the plant. If harvesting, focus your intention on your ancestral line, which has brought you to this moment and the transformational power of the henbane.

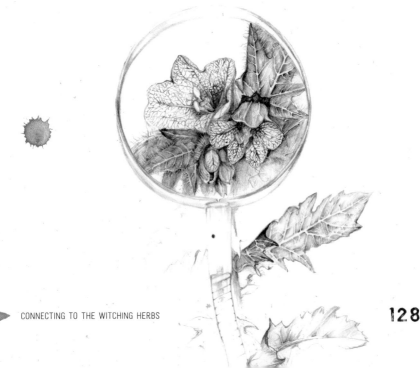

HONOUR YOUR ANCESTORS WITH HENBANE

As with datura, the seeds of henbane are extremely active and powerful. In this simple ritual, you can use henbane as a way of honouring your ancestors.

Steps:

1. Prepare to plant your henbane seeds in the spring after the last frost has past.
2. To potentize your henbane, place your seeds in a crystal bowl filled with spring water on your altar and then leave it to absorb the lunar rays overnight.
3. Decorate a pot with images of the ancestor you want to honour, or with writing about them. In this way, you will literally be growing the herb in honour of them and to connect with them.
4. Plant your seeds in your pot, with good-quality organic potting compost. You may wish to sow them on a Thursday (astrologically ruled by Jupiter), Saturday (ruled by Saturn) or Sunday (ruled by the sun) to honour the cosmic forces associated with this plant and call in the respective deities.
5. Once planted, water them well and cover the pot with either glass or cling film to keep the moisture in. As the seeds are germinating it is important to keep moisture in the soil.

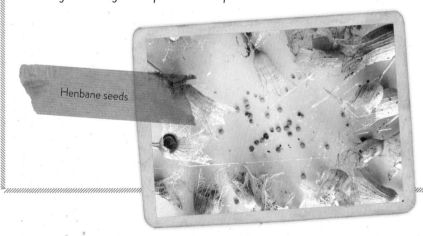

Henbane seeds

HENBANE IN HEALING

Henbane has many applications – from folk remedies to modern-day medicine. We like to dry the leaves and flowers for creation of an oil, although usually only the leaves are picked and utilized for tincturing within clinical medical herbalism in the UK (see page 135). In particular, we like to turn the plant into a flower essence. This potent remedy is especially useful in aiding connections with other realms, the underworld and of course the ancestors who reside there. Its healing energy can be used for cleansing ancestral lines and for laying to rest traumas that seep through the generations.

Other healing uses for henbane have been rather surprising – from dentistry to sedation. In his *Herball* of 1597, the English herbalist and botanist John Gerald writes about the multitudinous virtues of the plant:

> To wash the feet in the decoction of Henbane causeth sleep; or given in a clyster it doth the same; and also the often smelling to the flowers.
>
> The leaves, seed, and juice taken inwardly causeth an unquiet sleep like unto the sleep of drunkenness, which continueth long, and is deadly to the party.
>
> The root boiled with vinegar, and the same holden hot in the mouth, easeth the pain of the teeth. The seed is used by mountebank tooth-drawers which run about the country, for to cause worms come forth of men's teeth, by burning it in a chafing-dish with coals, the party holding his mouth over the fume thereof: but some crafty companions to gain money convey small lute strings into the water, persuading the patient that those small creeping beasts came out of his mouth or other parts which he intended to ease.

The Doctrine of Signatures

Writing in the 16th century, the Swiss–German physician and alchemist Paracelsus noted that: "Nature marks each growth ... according to its curative benefit." The doctrine of signatures was by then an ancient ideology, according to which plants, fruits and vegetables have an imprint marked upon them by Spirit, which offers clues as to their uses.

The doctrine dates to at least the times of the Roman naturalist Pliny the Elder (*c*. 20–79 CE), the Greek physician Dioscorides (*c*. 40–90 CE) and the Greek surgeon and philosopher Galen (*c*. 129–210 CE). However, it is hard to pinpoint the exact originate of the theory, as the concept will have been followed by numerous cultures and healing traditions. Wherever peoples have made detailed observations of nature, a version of the system can be found: traditional Chinese medicine, to Native American herbalism, Ayurveda and African herbalism.

The doctrine was an important part of folk medicine and often associated with herbalists and the wise healers. According to it, plants that work their healing ways on certain organs and body parts, like the blood or the eye, show a certain "signature" by resembling the thing they treat. The leaves of lungwort (*Pulmonaria officinalis*) look like diseased lungs and so were used to treat lung diseases; the structure of the eyebright flower (*Euphrasia officinalis*) resembles an eye so the plant was used to treat eye conditions. The Cherokee still take common purslane's stalks, which resemble worms, to treat worms in humans to great effect.

The seed heads of henbane look like a piece of jawbone complete with a row of teeth, so it was perhaps inevitable that the plant should have been used in dentistry.

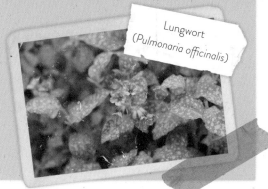

Lungwort (*Pulmonaria officinalis*)

DENTISTRY

Throughout time and cultures, henbane has been associated with dental procedures, signified by the jawbone shape of the henbane seed head.

As most of us are aware, controlling pain is critical to many dental procedures. With pain-dulling practices starting as early as 2250 BCE, the evolution of dental anaesthesia has come a long way to help make the most invasive oral procedures possible. The oldest record of this practice is found on an ancient Babylonian clay tablet where it is written that a mixture of henbane seed and gum mastic were mixed together to form a type of "cement" and applied for the pain of dental cavities. (It'd be worth asking for this next time a visit to the dentist is in order!)

In medieval medicine, henbane seeds were heated over coal or charcoal until they produced fumes which were then inhaled as a painkilling treatment for toothache. Another "cure" involved burning a mixture of frankincense, henbane and onion seeds. There was a belief that worms lived inside teeth and were responsible for any pain, so the patient funnelled the smoke toward the affected tooth. The worms supposedly wriggled out of the tooth and the pain disappeared – wishful thinking maybe but interesting to wonder whether the idea of worms could have been an early grasp of the existence of bacteria eating the gums and teeth.

As well as the medicinal applications of burning the plant that they call *Sakaran*, a name which translates as "the drunken one", the leaves and seeds of henbane are still smoked recreationally among Arabic-speaking nomadic Bedouin peoples. This custom has existed for centuries; perhaps an unexpectedly pleasant visit to the dentist led to their exploring the more recreational effects of the smoke.

THE SEDATIVE PROPERTIES OF HENBANE

As well as for pain relief during dental work, henbane has been deployed for other surgical procedures. The herb was used most often as an alternative to opium to sedate patients. Compared with opium, henbane arguably creates fewer negative side effects since it does not cause constipation, which is an issue with opium use. Henbane is extremely effective when applied to induce sleep and to calm unbalanced nerves.

ANCIENT ANAESTHESIA AND THE NIGHTSHADES

The nightshade family has been used anaesthetically for thousands of years – especially henbane. Evidence of pre-modern anaesthetic use for surgery suggests that the healers of old used both Solanaceae and Papaerveraceae (poppy) family plants in their recipes. The sedative properties of opium, extracted from poppy seed pods, were used in ancient Greece and Rome.

Our modern surgery has been developed from an ancient art. During the 6th century BCE, an Indian physician named Sushruta – widely regarded in India as the father of surgery – wrote one of the world's earliest works on medicine and surgery. The *Sushruta Samhita* documented over 1,000 medical conditions, along with the use of hundreds of medicinal plants and instructions for performing scores of surgical procedures, including three types of skin grafts and reconstruction of the nose.

Humans have always needed to be operated on in one way or another for procedures such as teeth extraction, setting bones and the removal of alien materials. Many of us may believe that in the past a patient would just have had to grin and bear it, and movies often show patients biting on bits of wood during operations. There is, however, plenty of evidence that surgery was far more sophisticated and that we used anaesthesia much earlier in our history than is generally imagined. Descriptions of anaesthetics based on mixtures of medicinal herbs have been found in manuscripts dating from before Roman times, until well into the Middle Ages.

Regions of southern Europe where certain sedative herbs grew abundantly are particularly rich in manuscripts written by monks documenting the use of herbs for anaesthesia. One text dating from 800 CE, from the Benedictine monastery at Monte Cassino in southern Italy, outlines a mixture of opium, henbane, mulberry juice, lettuce, hemlock, mandragora and ivy.

Soporific sponges were favoured in the Middle Ages for pain relief, soaked in plant formulas and held over the mouth and under the nostrils to send the patient into a stupor. The four ingredients commonly used in Europe in the earliest soporific sponge were opium, hemlock, mandrake and henbane. There are records from medieval England that suggest a drink called dwale, used for pain relief, was made from belladonna and henbane among other herbs.

Seventeenth-century records show that henbane was one of the most popular herbs of choice for pain relief and sedation during amputation. Recently dozens of henbane seeds were discovered in clay during the excavations of Tolbooth Jail in Stirling, Scotland. These were found in the medical area of the prison and are thought to be stock for surgery-related pain relief.

The use of the nightshade family for anaesthesia has continued down the centuries. Here is an extract from the article "A substitute for the Vapour of Ether to annul Sensation during Operations" in *The Lancet* medical journal from 1847:

> At midsummer, when vegetation is at its height, *Solanum nigrum, Hyoscyamus niger, Cicuta minor, Datura stramonium*, and *Lactuca virosa* are gathered, and a sponge is plunged into their juice freshly expressed. The sponge is then dried in the sun, the process of dipping and drying is repeated two or three times, and the sponge is then laid up in a dry place. When the sponge is required for use, it is soaked for a short time in hot water; afterwards it is placed under the nose of the person to be operated upon, who is quickly plunged into sleep. The operation may then be proceeded with without any fear that the patient has any sensation of pain. He is readily aroused from the stupor by a rag dipped in vinegar, and placed to his nose.

The modern use of omnopon (from opium poppy) and scopolamine (from the Solanaceae plants) show the value of these herbs in anaesthesia. Poppy heads and mandrake roots feature on the coat of arms of today's Association of Anaesthetists.

Laudanum

One of the main ingredients in a recipe developed by 16th-century physician Paracelsus for the famed opiate concoction laudanum was henbane root.

Many an artist and poet took creative inspiration from laudanum – Bram Stoker, Charles Dickens, Dante, Shelley and Lord Byron among them. One evocative work said to have been inspired by the drug is the poem "Kubla Khan" by the Romantic poet Samuel Taylor Coleridge, in which he describes a place "as holy and enchanted / As e'er beneath a waning moon was haunted / By woman wailing for her demon-lover".

HENBANE IN CLINICAL HERBALISM

In modern clinical herbalism, *Hyoscyamus niger* tincture is made from the leaves in a 1 in 10 preparation. This means that 1 part of leaves is put with 9 parts alcohol to create the tincture. This is a relatively low amount of herb for a tincture creation and reflects the strength of the alkaloids present (see Chapter 5). With certain other herbal preparations such as chamomile, for example, you would make a 1 in 2 or even 1 in 1, as there are very different, arguably less potent compounds involved.

The recommended maximum dosage of the henbane tincture of a 1 in 10 preparation is 5 to 20ml (1 to 4 tsp) per week, and around 1 to 3ml (20 to 60 drops) a day. Double the amount is permitted for dosing with henbane than for either datura or belladonna. This gives an indication as to the less problematic dosing and potential for overdose with henbane than the other two plants. This is because henbane contains higher amounts of the alkaloid hyoscyamine than belladonna and datura. As a result henbane causes a more overtly tranquillizing or narcotic action in comparison to its relatives.

The herb is indicated whenever there are intense spasms in the body that can cause tension, cramping and pain. Henbane is a specific herb used for menstrual cramps and gastrointestinal or bladder spasms because of this powerful antispasmodic action.

135

Medical herbalist Latifa Pelletirer-Ahmed, a peer of ours, harvests and makes her own henbane tincture, which she uses regularly for the treatment of menstrual cramps. She states that a dosage of 3 to 5ml is required of a 1:10 tincture of the leaves, the effect of which lasts for two to three hours but is diminished by eating. This is actually a pretty high dose over the course of a day, but Latifa usually sees it providing good results in about 10 to 20 minutes. She learned about it from another herbalist who uses belladonna in this way. Henbane grows as weeds where she lives so it's easy for her to find and harvest them. She has used the herb personally and on friends and family, who confirm its efficacy.

Herbalist Anne Cheshire explained to us that she has used henbane tincture with several patients, all of whom were prescribed a couple of drops under their tongues when experiencing bladder or urethral spasms. She has witnessed their immediate relief. Anne describes henbane medicine as having a lateral, spreading energy to it, and prescribes it to her patients who are too vertical in their energy – which she describes as being single-minded, overly focused and/or reluctant to engage in physical living, among other indicators. She sees henbane as broadening people's perspective in a different way to belladonna, which she regards as being very vertical in its energy, something that can be useful if the patient is scared stiff of opening up.

There are different applications of henbane that can be employed, and we have experimented with several recipes including ointment-based applications, which are extremely effective for treating dragging cramps and lower back ache. Henbane can also be applied as an external preparation for arthritis and joint pains. There is an Indian recipe for a pain-reliving oil that harnesses the medicine of the seeds, which are warmed with sesame oil and then rubbed on affected areas.

Henbane medicine can be employed for treating delirium, restlessness, excitability and insomnia. It is also indicated for motion sickness and Ménière's disease.

PSYCHOTROPIC THERAPEUTIC APPLICATION

As we have seen, henbane has associations with the celebration of death and therefore life. We can call on the powers of henbane's spirit energetically and metaphorically to walk toward the end of life with individuals, and to enter into a state of acceptance through recounting stories, untangling stuck emotions or regrets. This is prescribed in a psychotherapeutic way with specific exercises and processes to accompany its application.

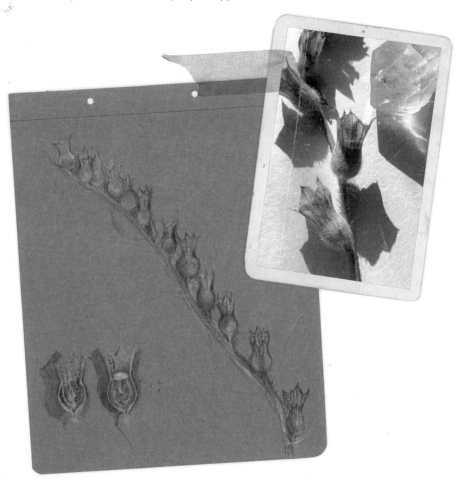

HENBANE EARTH MAGIC

There are particular auspicious times to practise magical work with henbane and especially for work with contacting the dead. Because henbane is deeply associated with the underworld and passing to other realms, the dark moon is a perfect lunar phase for henbane-assisted work – a time for introspection and delving deep. Similarly, a new moon occurring in an astrological Water sign such as Aquarius, Scorpio or Pisces will also enhance this reflective and emotive work. Water holds the memory of what is whispered to it, and of what has been held in it; the great oceans of the Earth tell the story of evolution, of life and of destruction. The astrological Water signs likewise keep us in touch with our emotional body and, as we do this work, emotions may surface.

In Greek mythology, the River Styx, the largest of all five of the mythological rivers, formed the boundary between the Earth and the underworld, flowing seven times in a spiral between the two realms of the living and the dead. It was also a river with great powers of immortality. Named after a daughter of the god Oceanus, the Styx was the river in which Achilles was dipped by his mother to give him his invincible powers – except for his vulnerable heel where he was held during his immersion.

It is said that those who were heading toward death were gifted henbane wreaths to wear. There are many theories as to why this might be – perhaps to forget the waking life you had before, or to bring about acceptance of what had happened and therefore the ability to pass over. As mentioned, henbane is one of the nightshades you can use in work with people who are transiting toward death to help support the re-telling of their life stories, and help them tie up loose ends.

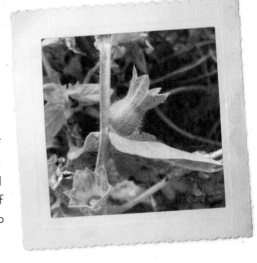

WREATH MAKING

Henbane connects us to a liminal state that enables the free flow of creativity and the letting go of anything negative that might be holding us back. The creation of a wreath will assist your connection to the ancestors in your magical practices.

You will need:

* long, thin lengths of ivy with the leaves left on, or another non-irritant bendy plant such as willow whips, honeysuckle or hazel
* dried henbane flowers on their stems
* twine or wire
* white ribbon

Steps:

1. Wrap the ivy, willow, honeysuckle or hazel around your head; then weave it into itself so that it holds as a circle. If you are using wire to form the base, wind ivy around it to add volume to the wreath.
2. When the hoop fits comfortably on your head, take the dried henbane flowers and poke them into the structure of your wreath, using the twine or wire to secure them in place.
3. Take your ribbon and wrap it around your wreath, tying three knots while repeating your intention.
4. When you are happy with your wreath, leave it on your altar space, ready for use when you carry out ancestral connection work.

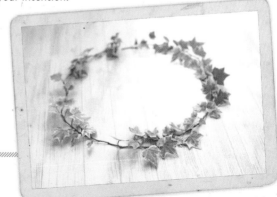

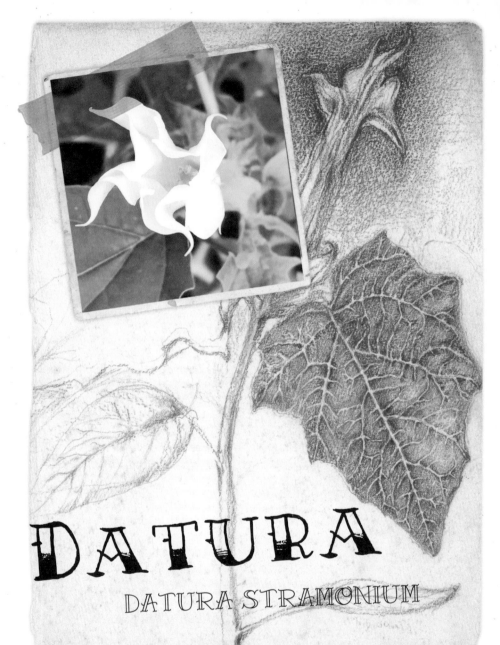

DATURA

DATURA STRAMONIUM

DATURA STRAMONIUM

- 7 -

DATURA

SHAPESHIFTING SEDUCTRESS

atura has a shadowy history and a tale that needs to be told. As we will see, it has long been associated with the wildness of werewolves, as many psychonauts have found in their journeys to other realms. In our experience with this plant, there is particularly deep internal medicine at work, where introspection is gifted. Datura has a dark nature that takes us to the hidden places, including those that might be thought of as lurking in the shadowy recesses of our subconscious patterns and behaviours. In taking us to these places, datura shines awareness on them like the full moon in the depths of the night. We will be looking at the healing actions associated with this revered plant medicine to help us to understand this much demonized and greatly feared herb.

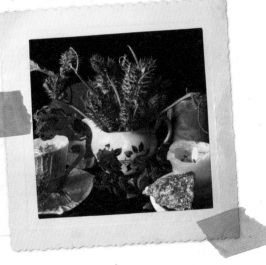

Latin name
Datura stramonium

Common names
Datura, thorn apple, insane herb, jimsonweed, moonflower, angel's trumpet, dotter (Dutch), Shiva's plant, kechu-booh (Egyptian)

Astrological rulers
Moon, Saturn

Actions
Internal application: anodyne, anti-anxiety, antiasthmatic, anticholinergic, anti-nausea, antidepressant, antisialagogue, antispasmodic, aphrodisiac, euphoric, sedative, narcotic, and soporific; topical applications: analgesic, anti-inflammatory, antispasmodic

Etymology
The plant's name, datura, derives from the early Sanskrit names of *dustura* or *dahatura*, meaning "divine inebriation". The most commonly found species of datura in the UK is *Datura stramonium*. *Stramonium* originated from the Greek word *strychnos*, which means nightshade or deadly, and "mankos" meaning "mad". In classical times the Greeks used the word *strychnos* to describe several plants that contained the powerful tropane alkaloids.

Distribution
Datura species are said to originate from the dry, temperate and subtropical areas of Mexico and other countries on the Americas, but there is evidence to suggest the herb travelled to Europe from an easterly direction, possibly by Gypsies and travelling traders. It grows across the world except for in very cold climates such as the Antarctic. The herbalist John Gerard (*c*.1545–1612) claimed to have distributed the first seeds of *D. stramonium* in England, but we cannot be sure that this is true. This plant would have been in many hands, and its possession by nomadic and common country folk would simply not have been documented.

GETTING TO KNOW DATURA

Datura is completely unforgettable with her strong, sticky stems, deep green leaves, elegant flowers and spiky seedpods. A vespertine beauty, she gradually became integrated into the sophisticated cultural belief systems associated with magic and witchcraft. Datura plants usually grow as gloriously eye-catching herbaceous annuals, or perennials. They are strikingly characterized by their large, beautifully coloured (white to pinkish) trumpet-like flowers, which typically exude a fragrant odour nocturnally. They also bear walnut-sized seed capsules covered with spiky thorns; hence their English common name "thorn apple" and the German *Stechapfel*.

Flowering at night, datura tricks the moths with her luminous, moon-like appearance and sweet smell to pollinate her trumpets. The heady, rich scent is notably more powerful at night when the plant prepares to attract her pollinators.

After flowering, the most magnificent spiky seed pods (also known as thorn apples) start to form before cracking open to reveal hundreds of black seeds in each pod. This contrast between the bright white inflorescence of the flowers and the jet-black seeds of the *stramonium* species is noteworthy.

While *Datura stramonium*, *Datura inoxia* and *Datura metel* are the most commonly found three varieties, we will be focusing on *D. stramonium* that grows in many parts of the world.

MEET DATURA THE DIVA

The Diva Datura is a night-walking age-shifter who can turn from a fertile and sexy seductress to a wise grandmother crone – still sultry and stunningly beautiful. This lady is a witch, breathing life and passion into creativity. Diva is a jazz singer with a husky rich voice. She weaves magic on her every breath, each note inviting attention. She never sees the light of day as she spends each and every night singing her music to a crowd of adoring fans. She is busty, hippy, deliciously curvaceous and attracts loyal followers. She sits in the bright spotlight with the dark all around her, chain-smoking, her eyes missing nothing.

KEY THEMES FOR DATURA

One word that can be associated with datura is that of "shapeshifting" as this plant gives us the ability to shift smoothly into new skin, shedding the old.

In large doses, datura can remove the concept of time; minutes, hours and even days can be lost as if time no longer exists in a linear fashion. In small doses, datura can bring a sense of stopping time in order to reflect and understand why we have irrational feelings, fears or anxieties. This can gift ways of unpacking and leaving old patterns behind – shapeshifting away from buried pain into a sense of freedom.

* For understanding different aspects of the self, delving deep, introspection
* Shapeshifting
* Facing fears
* Embodying various roles in life
* Untangling old patterns, delving deep
* Self-revelation – knowing yourself
* Introspection
* Empowerment
* Light and dark
* Breathing deeply, remaining open to life by embracing darkness

DATURA CULTIVATION

Datura stramonium is an annual, meaning its whole life cycle happens in a year. It flowers, creates seed and then dies, leaving a woody skeleton behind.

Datura is the easiest of our three nightshades to grow. The seeds are about the size of a dress-maker's pinhead but more flattened. Germination of the dark, black, kidney-shaped seeds seems to be pretty swift, at around seven to ten days. Although the plant prefers rich, well-drained soil, she tolerates a variety of soil types. Datura naturally prefers light and open space; we've found her growing just as well from the cracks in a yard with little nutrient intake as at the edge of crop fields.

The large, irregularly undulating leaves are situated in freely bracing stems. They are extremely sticky and just a brush of the finger leaves a bitter exudate on the tip. Each leaf branch hosts a majestic white trumpet flower that uncurls, releasing an intoxicating perfume, particularly at night. The flowers become spiked thorn-apple seed pods which dry and start to split, releasing hundreds of the dark seeds.

Datura need to be watered regularly while the plant is establishing. If planted outdoors, which she tolerates very well, and once matured, the plant does not require watering as it seeks hydration deeply in the soil with the help of its long taproot.

Slugs love to demolish young datura plants so they need to be protected well during early growth. Slugs obviously have very different nervous system responses to humans, the amount of datura that one slug can consume far outweighs that of a human without seeing serious consequences.

Datura plants are considered invasive weeds in much of the world as they can easily spread if grown in favourable conditions.

HARVESTING DATURA

It is suggested by the English herbalist Maude Grieves (1858–1941) that – unlike with many other herbs – it's best to harvest the leaves of datura when the plant is in full bloom. Upon observation of the plant, we can see that the leaves do hold their colour and vibrancy even when the plant is blossoming, so it is best to harvest them before the seed pods start to develop, when the edges of the leaves start to turn yellow. These can then be dried or tinctured for medicinal and magical applications.

The trumpet-like flowers are best picked around the full moon for a potent flower essence that has the energy of shining a light in deep, dark spaces, offering illumination of emotional hooks and the power to blow a fresh breeze through them, clearing and providing a new perspective.

The multitude of seeds held in each pod of *Datura stramonium* go a dark black colour when ready and burst out. To dry the seeds, sparsely lay them out on a piece of cardboard or paper and leave in a well-aerated space for a few days.

They can be stored, once properly dried, until the following spring. They need to be efficiently dried because they tend to go mouldy if any moisture is left in them. The thorn-apple seed pod is charged with the qualities of fierce protection, longevity and survival. In one experiment seeds stored for 40 years still had a germination rate of over 90 per cent.

THE HISTORY OF DATURA

Though datura does not seem to have been popularly used in Europe the way belladonna and henbane were, it is clear that in the British Isles, some Anglo-Saxon leeches (medicinal practitioners) certainly knew how to use it. The plant appears several times in the 4th-century *Herbarium*, where the herb is written about in mixtures for the treatment of impetigo, pimples, headache, stomach inflammation, hard swellings and earache.

Whatever its origins, datura appears to have played an important role as a power plant globally, and is mentioned in texts from Africa, Asia and the Americas – in fact from almost every inhabitable landmass for many years. Throughout the world, the herb has been and still is particularly valued for its ability to induce visionary dreams, to help in foretelling the future, for initiation ceremonies and to reveal the causes of disease and misfortune.

Datura has been highly revered in societies whose medical paradigm differs from the Western biomedical system in Europe. References to the sacred uses of *datura* (specifically *D. metel*) exist in many records from India, China and Mexico.

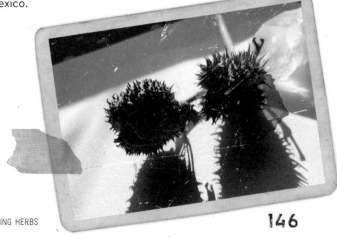

INDIA

India has lots of rich folklore about datura. One myth recounts how datura grew where a pair of underworld twins resided, who were famed for their sleep-inducing powers. There is another myth that the feared and revered datura plant originally grew out of Lord Shiva's chest.

This mysterious sexy diva plant is written about in the much-famed Indian text the *Kama Sutra* (c. 4th century CE). It is written that if a man anoints his *lingam* (phallus) with a mixture of the powders of *dhatturaka* (datura), *pippali* (long pepper), *maricha* (black pepper) and *madhu* (honey), and engages in sexual union with a woman, he makes her subject to his will. This sounds messy to be honest and just a tad too dominating for our liking, but much can be lost in translation! We know only too well about the aphrodisiac nature of datura; this lusty lady is a serious turn-on.

A remedy of the powdered seeds can be mixed with butter and ingested orally for impotence or applied topically to invigorate the male genitalia. Dr Bhakta Prasad Gaire is a researcher from India who had a very powerful experience over three days as a child after ingesting datura seeds out of hunger while waiting for his mother to return home. This experience led him to study datura in more depth and he writes about a datura butter that starts with boiled datura milk. To make it he used 15 ripe fruits (seeds and all), boiled gently with 8 litres (14 pints) of cow's milk. The datura-infused milk is made into a curd, which is then churned to make a medicinal butter. This butter can be rubbed into the penis and spine to treat impotence.

Datura leaves and seeds are mixed with *ganja* (*Cannabis indica* L.) and smoked by *sadhus* (holy men). As in many other parts of the world, the dried leaves of the datura are smoked widely for the relief of asthmatic symptoms.

While in India, we came across folk who were given biscuits laced with what they believed to be datura on a train before losing their memory and being robbed. We also encountered a woman who lived in a cave at night and huddled by a bridge in the daytime, who was said to have lost her way from datura ingestion. These are stark reminders of the flip side of these powerful revered plants and a good reminder to respect the herbs and their potency.

CHINA

Taoist legend refers to datura as *Man-t'o-lo* – "the flower of one of the pole stars". The polar region of the sky was particularly important for the ancient and medieval Chinese as it was said to mirror the authority of the emperor, and was highly regarded because of its prime position. Similar to India, *Datura stramonium* and *Cannabis sativa* were combined in Chinese medicine. Ancient medical Chinese texts state that if consumed in equal quantities, these two herbs would produce such a powerful anaesthesia that surgery could be performed.

THE AMERICAS

There is a long and varied history of datura use all over the American continent – from the ancient Aztecs to the Indigenous peoples of Canada.

Among the Navajo, the dried roots were chewed in ceremonies as a febrifuge (to stop fever), while a leaf infusion was used as a vulnerary (a wound-healing agent).

The Chumash of California used datura as an anaesthetic for bone setting, and to treat wounds, bruises and haemorrhoids. The herb was also important in initiation rituals to welcome the youth of the tribe into adulthood. To them, datura was the single most important medicinal plant. It was taken in a ritualistic framework and applied to seek support in the dream state and in contacting the ancestors, and was said to aid communication to spirit guides.

The Powhattans held "huskinawing", their term for puberty initiation rites held each spring for young males becoming braves. This ceremony of transition into manhood used datura alongside days spent in the wilderness. Many other tribes including the Zunis, Paiutes and Walapais used the plant for similar purposes.

CENTRAL AND SOUTH AMERICAN REGIONS

The ancient Aztecs of Mexico also made use of datura, which they referred to as *ololluhqui*, meaning "the magic plant". They utilized datura for treating a host of diseases, including paralysis. It was possibly given as an external preparation and also applied as an ointment for cuts or wounds.

Coming-of-Age Rituals

For those of us who grew up in Europe, while our own adolescent rites of passage might have been pretty intense, they weren't held by the wider community; we had to create them ourselves with our peers. The results were far from sacred as all too often we simply searched for any intoxicants we could find, in somewhat nihilistic "rituals" designed to get off our heads! Gateways into the realm of adulthood might have included cheap cider, magic mushrooms, a variety of grass and cannabis resins, LSD, copious amounts of ecstasy – and that was just to start with! Our ritualistic "wilderness" was often an abandoned warehouse, forests and disused waste grounds, where we'd set up sound systems and danced to repetitive beats. We've probably all fallen into a fair few ditches over the years – ditches that we had to climb out of, literally and metaphorically.

Rituals are so important to societies and to our understanding of our place in the tribe or community. In the modern era teenagers are commonly feared, with the media demonizing them. How different would it be for the whole neighbourhood to watch over and design rituals for youth to grow into? To allow them space but also a net of support as they explore what it means to grow into adulthood?

The plant's narcotic effects were employed by the priests to communicate with spirits. Cigars were rolled with datura's leaves or the seeds were eaten, which would cause visions and stimulate people to dance, laugh, weep, sleep or tell oracular prophecies. The seeds were considered sacred and kept on altars or in secret boxes and sacrificial offerings were made to them. We love the practice of bringing seeds to the altar and potentizing them before planting. You will often find little boxes of seeds on our altar spaces, and we encourage you to do this too.

In present-day Mexico, datura is called *toloache*, which translates as "reverential". In a low dose, *toloache* operates as a pain reliever. In Mexican *brujeria* (or witchcraft), modern-day medicine people make love potions from this revered herb. Many markets that sell magical powders and potions will carry *toloache* products. Folklore suggests that mixing it into the food or tobacco of the person you desire will make them fall in love with you.

Amazonian tribes sometimes integrated datura into ayahuasca brews under the name *toé*. Like ayahuasca ceremonies, stand-alone *toé* ceremonies have been practised by Amazonian communities for generations. Called dream journeys, these datura-focused experiences are used to enhance the power of divination and vision.

There are common threads here of sacred use for visions, pain relief and as an aphrodisiac. All powerful applications are indicative of the herb's potency.

NORTH AMERICAN REGION

Commonly called "jimsonweed" in North America, this name is a corruption of "Jamestown weed" – and a reference to its mass consumption and the subsequent "trip" experienced by a band of English colonizers.

In 1676, the settlers in Jamestown took matters into their own hands when they felt their governor was not doing enough to protect them from the area's Native American tribes. Led by Nathaniel Bacon, the settlers decided to become vigilantes and attack the Native Americans in the area. Bacon's men violently assaulted and murdered people from several tribes, provoking a potential war. In response, the governor sent in troops to put down the uprising, which is now known as Bacon's Rebellion. The soldiers did eventually suppress the rebellion, but only after the rebels burned down Jamestown and a number of the governor's soldiers became unwitting guinea pigs in demonstrating the powerful effects of "Jamestown weed". Writing in 1705, American historian Robert Beverley, Jr (1667–1722) described the mass hallucination that took place:

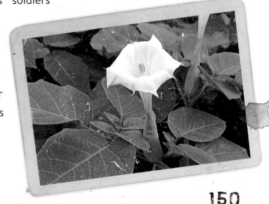

The James-Town Weed (which resembles the Thorny Apple of Peru, and I take to be the plant so call'd) is supposed to be one of the greatest coolers in the world. This being an early plant, was gather'd very young for a boil'd salad, by some of the soldiers sent thither to quell the rebellion of Bacon (1676); and some of them ate plentifully of it, the effect of which was a very pleasant comedy, for they turned natural fools upon it for several days: one would blow up a feather in the air; another would dart straws at it with much fury; and another, stark naked, was sitting up in a corner like a monkey, grinning and making mows at them; a fourth would fondly kiss and paw his companions, and sneer in their faces with a countenance more antic than any in a Dutch droll.

In this frantic condition they were confined, lest they should, in their folly, destroy themselves – though it was observed that all their actions were full of innocence and good nature. Indeed, they were not very cleanly; for they would have wallowed in their own excrements, if they had not been prevented. A thousand such simple tricks they played, and after eleven days returned themselves again, not remembering anything that had passed.

EUROPE

Historical information about datura is hard to ascertain in Europe. There are very few accounts and much of what we do have is based on the premise that these herbs were utilized for malevolent "witchcraft" – the result of a very specific time and a very specific viewpoint.

Michael Harner is an anthropologist famed for his work documenting indigenous medicine practices. His book, *The Way of the Shaman*, published in 1980, was widely read and has been associated with the popularization of so-called "shamanic practices". As we have touched upon earlier in this book, these have since proliferated massively, with questionable results.

The term "shamanism" originally comes from the Manchu-Tungus' word *šaman*, which in turn is formed from the word *ša*, meaning "to know". Thus, a shaman is literally "one who knows". The Maanchu-Tungus is a vast region that stretches from northern China across Mongolia to the northern boundary of Russia. There are between 15 and 20 languages spoken in the region.

In his earlier book, *Hallucinogens and Shamanism* (1973), Harner writes of practices in Europe during the Middle Ages involving the use of a broom to apply psychotropic salves to sensitive vaginal membranes. Harner was not a historian but a popular writer and anthropologist in amongst the 70s crowd with interest in reaching altered states. The historical veracity of the resulting image of the witch flying on her broomstick has been disputed by modern historian Thomas Hatsis, who has not found any reference to the ointment being applied by this method in his research. However, we believe that various wooden implements would have naturally been used by women to apply a psychotropic lube – and a broom handle seems as good as any! We can tell you that modern-day witches are very much pleasuring themselves with broom handles and flying free on the sabbats. But back to datura ...

We have already encountered the herbalist John Gerard at the start of this chapter. The herbalist had a physic garden in London and grew the plant from seeds he gathered in Constantinople. He declares:

> The juice of Thornapple, boiled with hog's grease, cureth all inflammations whatsoever, all manner of burnings and scaldings, as well as of fire, water, boiling lead, gunpowder, as that which comes by lightning and that, in very short time, as myself have found in daily practice, to my great credit and profit.

Although it is unclear how he came to know the uses of datura, Gerard was able to heal scalds and burns with his hog's grease-datura ointment. Interestingly, in his original herbal housed in the Wellcome Library, London, he swaps the identities of the two species of datura he features, perhaps by mistake, labelling *D. stramonium* as *D. inoxia* and vice versa.

DATURA'S MYTHOLOGY – WEREWOLVES AND ZOMBIES

The werewolf has become so embedded in our collective psyche that unearthing the root of the myth is difficult. As mentioned in Chapter 5, there are suggestions that datura intoxication could be linked to the werewolf myth. Reports from hospital rooms in the 1970s, when datura intoxication was at its modern height, record apparent sightings of werewolf-like creatures. Datura can make people around you appear to be covered in hair, and it has even been reported that it can make goats walk on their back legs upright when under the influence! We know that datura cuts off learned behaviours, so there is a chance that it reveals mythological creatures from our collective psyche, such as the werewolf.

Feelings of morphing into wolves – our bodies growing hairier and hands turning into paws – are common when under the influence of datura, especially when imbibed during the luminous full moon. Because of its werewolf mythology, this plant interweaves in our minds with little red riding hood, the innocent making her way through the woods, where there is much peril and distraction.

As well as werewolves, datura is linked to another fearsome creature of the collective imagination: the zombie. Many of us have grown up with classic zombie stories and movies such as *Night of the Living Dead*. Zombies are animated corpses with a ravenous appetites and as soon as they bite you, you are infected with the loathsome zombie virus.

The myth of the zombie might be connected to the datura plant. Zombie folklore is sometimes attributed to Haiti, where it has been around for centuries. The zombie story possibly originates in the 17th century when West African enslaved peoples were brought in to work on Haiti's sugar cane plantations. It seems that this voodoo, candomble or mandinga custom began in Africa before being introduced to the Mediterranean and Indonesian islands, the Caribbean, and coming to the Americas with the atrocious slave trade. A Haitian name for the datura plant is *concombre zombi*, the "zombie's cucumber", and datura was one of the main plants used to induce what was termed "possession inebriation", which caused raptures of bodily frenzy during which conscious awareness was lost. Brutal conditions left the enslaved peoples longing for freedom. According to some reports, the life – or rather afterlife – of a zombie represented the horrific plight of slavery.

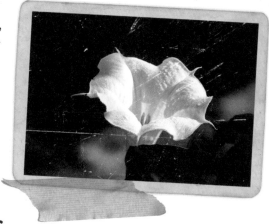

DATURA IN HEALING

During the course of connecting people with the subtitles of datura over the years, we have witnessed an extremely introspective response to the herb. Suddenly there is less chatter in the room and folk are more reserved or say less when we ask for feedback about their connection, feelings and physical symptoms with the plant. They often experience a sense of travelling inward. This contemplation and deep dive into the self can provide space in which to fully discover and explore our inner shadow lands.

Datura's connection with the moon speaks of the herb's ability to illuminate hidden aspects of our selves or parts that we could perhaps shed light on and feel more comfortable inhabiting. She brings illumination into the areas that we need to pay attention to. She takes us deep within ourselves in order to draw us out, open up and help us breathe in and accept all versions of ourselves.

Datura has the ability to expose us to the mysterious archetypal aspects of ourselves; she reveals hidden recesses and dredges up ancient tribulations your energetic line has experienced. Datura shows us where we struggle, where we hold fears and neuroses, and can offer us keys to let go and allow life to flow more easily. This relates to the psycho-therapeutic idea of the shadow places, those aspects we may not notice in day-to-day life but which affect our every reaction and how we show ourselves to the world; subconscious or hidden fears. Datura shines a bright white glow in our darkness, like the mistress of the night that she is. She is unafraid to explore what goes bump in the night!

SLEEP MEDICINE

Many cultures have applied datura mixed with other plants as a sleep aid. Two ancient Greek botanists living several centuries apart, Dioscorides and Theophrastus, both stated that datura was used as an *hypnotikon*, meaning a sleep-inducer. A recommended preparation was to soak the herb in wine. The *De Medicina* of the Roman encyclopaedist Cornelius Celsus (c. 25 BCE to 50 CE) records the sleep-inducing nature of the herb.

We have pondered the possible reasons for datura's application in insomnia, and deduced the following. It has been suggested that the cholinergic system in the brain (see page 101) is the regulator for serotonin-induced pathways of sleep. While serotonin has been widely established to initiate REM sleep, it looks like the neurotransmitter Acetylcholine (or ACh) has the role of ensuring that awareness is maintained while sleep is occurring. ACh thus keeps us vigilant while still asleep, protecting us from potential threats like fire. It enables a filtration of external sounds and other sensory indicators. If we interfere with the pathway of ACh as the tropane alkaloids do, could we then prevent sounds from the external environment interfering with our sleep patterns and dreams? We don't need to wake up if our partner stirs in bed but if there is a potential threat and the sounds are more alarming, do they require our conscious awareness? In the case of insomnia, where someone remains hypervigilant at night, interfering with this process could be enough to let them settle into a more deep and healing sleep.

DATURA IN CLINICAL HERBALISM

In modern clinical herbalism, *Datura stramonium* tincture is made from the plant's leaves, in a 1 in 10 preparation. As when using henbane, this means that 1 part of the leaves is put with 9 parts alcohol to create the tincture. This is a relatively low amount of herb for tincture creation and reflects the strength of the alkaloids present. The dosage of that preparation is 5 to 10ml (1 to 4 tsp) per week, around 1ml (20 drops) a day maximum.

Datura has a specific affinity for the lungs as a bronchodilator. When the lungs are restricted in asthma, there can be a lot of fear associated with the tight feeling and lack of available oxygen. This application works by the interference with the cholinergic system pathways and literally reduces the nerve pathway that causes the tightening of the lungs. It is an extremely effective anti-asthmatic herb but is used in combination with other herbs, and the dosage and effects are monitored regularly.

By opening up tight lungs, datura helps to expand and deepen the breath, to take in more oxygen and create a sense of engaging with, and filling up with, life. The breath represents life as the first thing we do after birth – inhale – and the last thing before death – exhale.

Herbalist Jean Dow told us that she has seen almost miraculous recoveries in the ability to breathe in lung cancer patients using datura tincture. Her first-ever patient had terminal lung cancer and the initial consultation only lasted 20 minutes because the patient couldn't breathe enough to speak. However, she prescribed datura and three weeks later the patient was able to engage in a full consultation for 90 minutes with no difficulty whatsoever. After being given four to eight weeks to live, her first patient lived for a further 22 months, and at 20 months was still able to go out and chop her own logs! Her ease of breathing was due to datura. This initial success with datura inspired Jean to specialize her work with more cancer patients.

During our training in the Archway Clinic of Herbal Medicine, London, clinical lecturer and experienced medical herbalist Graham Byde taught students how to prescribe datura in cases of asthma. The protocol he shared was for a datura-based combination for patients who were suffering an acute attack. Over the years we have developed our own version of this:

ASTHMA MIX

* 8ml (1.6 tsp) Datura stramonium – *datura*
* 50ml (3.4 tbsp) Plantago lanceloata – *plantain*
* 42ml (2.8 tbsp) Foeniculum vulgare – *fennel*

Directions:

1 to 3 drops every few minutes during any difficulty
with breathing and bronchial spasm.

This mix has provided beneficial relief in many people we have
treated suffering from asthma attacks. Careful monitoring
by an experienced herbalist during application will ensure
no side effects or interactions with other medication.

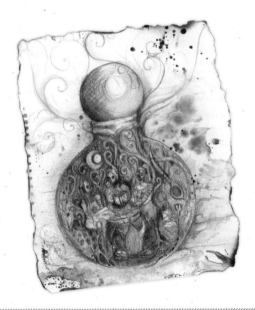

According to Byde, the 1968 Medicines Act in the UK led to a huge reduction in the use of these Solanaceae herbs among his peers. When the Medicines Act was introduced, the dosages of the Solanaceae herbs became recommended at much lower levels than many herbalists had been using beforehand. Byde suggests that the Solanaceae doses had become so restricted, many herbalists (himself included) simply ceased using them and opted to work with the herbs that had a higher dose allowance. As a comparison, asthma doses for *Lobelia inflata* and *Ephedra spp* (Indian and Chinese origin retrospectively) remained high under the restricted herb list. Lobelia has a maximum recommended dose of 200mg, which is four times that of the recommended dose of datura. Ephedra's recommended maximum dose is 600mg, which is 12 times that of datura. While Byde's is an interesting observation, we have had excellent results when using the recommended doses or much lower.

PSYCHOTROPIC THERAPEUTIC APPLICATIONS

A 1959 US publication suggests datura was used in criminology as a so-called "truth-drug" because it causes disturbed consciousness and a loss of short-term memory. This highlights that this plant can uncover truths within ourselves and reveal hidden aspects of our personalities for contemplation.

Unfortunately, many a trippy explorer has dabbled with datura without prior knowledge of dosage, resulting in their psycho-emotional edges being burned. There are many stories in the alternative party scene about folk returning from datura trips with tales of madness and whole lost days, void of any recollection. These stories have travelled throughout the alternative scene and spread fear into those experimenting with psychotropic plants. There is still a residue of fear surrounding the beautiful moonflower due to this association with death and madness.

Datura does not come without risks but heroic doses are not recommended with this beautiful and mysterious plant. She demands careful consideration, respect and small doses – and when this is offered she will gift inspiration and creativity. If drawing on the Diva Datura as a muse or to go deep into our psyche on journeys of inner exploration, it is important to use specific tools, exercises and affirmations alongside the herb, which is taken in small drop doses. Datura supports a sense of empowerment and self-belief, as we uncover the patterns that arise and potentially interfere with smooth-flowing daily life.

DATURA EARTH MAGIC

These are auspicious times for working magically with datura. Practising spell work and magic with datura is potentized around the illumination of the moon at its fullest. As drawing on the full energy of Fire will enhance the work still further, explore sexy spells using datura when the full moon is passing through the Fire signs of Aries, Leo or Sagittarius.

Datura is a wonderful temptress to draw on when exploring sex magic. Sex can act as a gateway to communication with the divine forces, and datura sports a tremendously sexual flower, intoxicating in the extreme – with one sniff capable of inducing the most erotic of imaginings and fantasies. The experience of sexual pleasure harnesses great power and when directed magically can be both healing and energizing. The sacred act of sex helps us to remember that our physical bodies have the ability to unleash incredible magnetic energy. We will be considering this in more detail in Chapter 16.

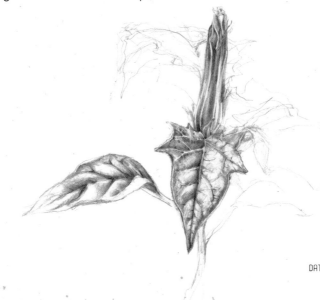

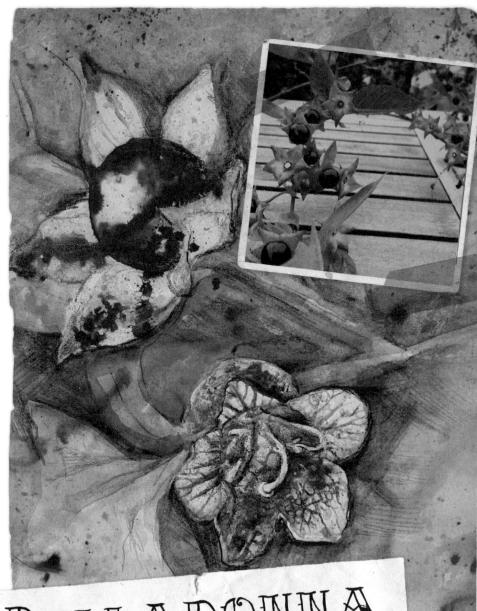

BELLADONNA

ATROPA BELLADONNA

– 8 –
BELLADONNA

FEARLESS FEMME FATALE

 native European power plant, Belladonna holds the keys to altered states of awareness and is a hugely beneficial physically active medicine. Since ancient times, this beauty has been famed for her poisonous properties and applications in witchcraft, sorcery and other forms of magic and medicine.

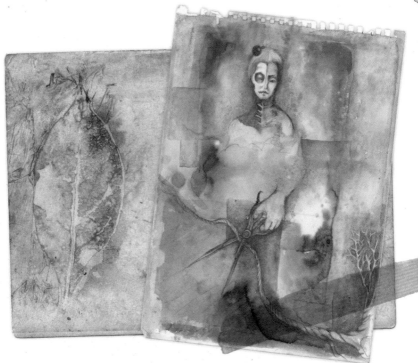

Latin name
Atropa belladonna

Astrological ruler
Saturn

Common names
Belladonna, deadly nightshade,
devil's cherry, divale, dwale,
banewort, devil's berries, death
cherries, beautiful death, devil's
herb, great morel, dwayberry

Actions
Analgesic, anodyne, anti-anxiety,
anti-inflammatory, anti-nausea,
antisialagogue, anticholinergic,
antidepressant, antispasmodic,
diuretic, mydriatic, narcotic,
sedative, soporific

Etymology
The names associated with this superstar plant are extremely
strong and evocative, such as "belladonna", from the Italian for
"beautiful lady". This name was given to the plant because the ladies
of Venice used *Atropa belladonna* as a cosmetic (see page 171).

Distribution
Native to temperate southern, Central and Eastern Europe, North
Africa, Turkey, Iran and the Caucasus. Naturalized in Britain and parts
of North America but considered a weed in other parts of the world.

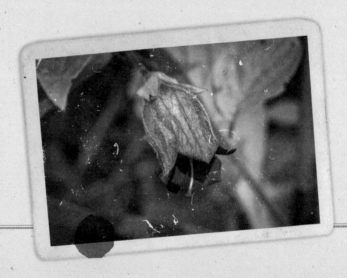

GETTING TO KNOW BELLADONNA

Belladonna's dark green foliage gives rise to hues of greens and purples in her aromatic blooms. Once these tubular flowers are pollinated they morph into the famous jet-black, shiny berries, often referred to as "devil's cherries". These mirrored spheres look like potential treats to the uninitiated and have even ended up in a pie or two! The taste of the berry is sweet and the vivid purple juice can look appetizing, especially as the plants can sometimes be found growing in hedgerows alongside blackberries, looking safe, delicious and tasty. It is possible that the term "devil's cherry" was coined to make children afraid of consuming the berries. Stories of summoning up Old Nick himself were told: "If you eat the devil's cherry, better be prepared to come face to face with the Devil ... "

Inside the obsidian balls are round, black seeds in gelatinous, deep purple fruit. Belladonna is a perennial; she will grow each year, returning from the same root stock. The leaves are oval-shaped, un-toothed and smooth — distinct from henbane and datura.

Atropa belladonna is the most famous of the perennial deadly nightshades but there are another three recognized, closely related species according to Kew Garden's botanical plant list: *Atropa acuminata* (Indian belladonna), *Atropa baetica* (one of Europe's rarest wildflowers) and *Atropa pallidiflora* (meaning pale flowers).

Over the years as we two Sistas became more attracted to this herb and her stories, intense magic started to seep into our consciousness, and she appeared to us in dreams as a mysterious witch. She serendipitously graced our garden with her presence, self-seeding in an untended bed, and we found ourselves making up our own stories about her ...

MEET BEATRIX NIGHTSHADE

The widow Beatrix Nightshade is an elegant woman in her sixties. She has thick, white hair with a deep purple streak, black eyes and dark pools reflecting within. She works as an undertaker, an eighth-generation mortician in her family. As a young woman, she didn't want to go into the family business, so she rebelled and studied the art of hairdressing. She is still requested by friends and family to get her scissors out occasionally to shape their coiffure.

She is the eldest of three daughters. Her sisters always came to her with their menstrual problems and now that they have all smoothly transitioned through the menopause with her expert care and secret potions, they send their daughters to her. A wonderful cool head in any stressful situation, Beatrix never loses her temper or gets hot and bothered.

She dances the tango to competitive levels and has a multitude of admirers. Anyone who gets close to her feels her passion and their hearts beat a little stronger. Her admirers are all slightly fearful of her, both attracted and repelled as there is gossip that she poisoned her ex-husband. He died young when they had only been married for three years and there is much speculation as to his passing.

KEY THEMES FOR BELLADONNA

With adulthood comes responsibility – and finding a job or a home, paying the rent or a mortgage, finding love and potentially breeding all have their own special set of pressures that create a serving of anxiety and fear. In adulthood, we experience the death of our care-free independence. We need to inhabit these new roles and new responsibilities without losing ourselves completely. Belladonna can help to celebrate the little deaths as we move through in life, and transition between our various roles, embracing and releasing any restrictions we might feel, cutting away all the baggage, freeing us from the binds and the worries that enslave our minds.

Belladonna's name has been associated with the attraction of a spidery, femme fatal. However, the deeper message of *Atropa belladonna* is that of the ravers, those wonton, wily Maenads; it is about finding our own wildness, a fabulous free dance and flow of momentum through the adventure of life. Being true to yourself will in turn attract the people who are meant to find you, to be part of your story.

We can use the energy of untamed wildness to free ourselves from the weight we carry and embrace our wild side, remaining true to our authentic nature:

* To be feral – permission to be wild and free
* Fierce grace
* Endings and new beginnings
* Shifting the sense of a fear of lack
* Cut away energetic shackles
* Releasing fears – link with Atropos
* Cutting ties to past relationships
* Clarity of mind
* Seeing clearly

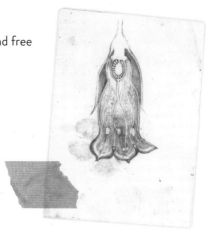

THE HISTORY OF BELLADONNA

As well as making women more attractive, belladonna has been associated with war, sex and death throughout history – another rock-star herb for the growing band!

Belladonna, like henbane, crops up in myths and legends of fighting and warring, and the plant is sacred to Bellona, the Roman goddess of war. Bellona was originally revered by the Sabine people, a tribe from central Italy. When the Sabines relocated to Rome they brought their important goddess Bellona along with them. The first recorded temple dedicated to Bellona was built around 300 BCE. The priests and priestesses of Bellona would consume belladonna berries before entering into a fervent and fanatical ritual space.

Some biblical scholars have postulated that various power plants hold answers as to how Christ could have withstood the barbaric torture and horrific pains of crucifixion. It is suggested that the "vinegar and gall" described in the Bible could have been a soporific, pain-relieving agent, to aid in a slightly more humane death. A variety of different recipes have been proposed, most containing a combination of belladonna, mandrake and wormwood mixed with other plant medicines.

In the medieval period, the Scottish lieutenant Macbeth laced beer with belladonna and somehow got it served to the invading troops. The King of England, Harold Harefoot, and his men drunk the poisoned brew and ended up feeling very odd, no doubt, and retreating. Macbeth eventually became King of Alba, a part of modern-day Scotland.

It's fascinating to discover that this ancient combat poison is still being deployed in modern conflicts, but nowadays not as a frenzy-inducing agent. Instead, the alkaloid atropine is employed in modern chemical warfare as an antidote to the nerve agent Sarin. It is successfully applied to counter the effects of the nerve agent, which causes fluid to build up in the respiratory organs. Atropine helps dry up secretions in the lungs.

BELLADONNA'S MYTHOLOGY - THE MAENADS

An early example of a psychotropic use of belladonna was at the Bacchanalia festivities of the Greco-Roman religious celebrations, where it was reputedly added to the wine. This celebration was in honour or Bacchus or Dionysus, the god of religious ecstasy and of the harvest, wine, intoxication and fertility.

The stories say that there were nymphs at these Dionysian orgies, and their appearance and behaviour is suggestive of belladonna intoxication. The female revellers were referred to as Maenads, so named from the ancient Greek for "raving, wild or frantic". These nymphs were depicted with dilated pupils and in a state of frantic wildness, dancing and cavorting in abandonment.

In a personal practice with this herb, you can feel this association, and call on belladonna's energetic medicine to welcome in and rediscover "the wild". We can abandon civility, completely letting go and becoming "raving mad", dancing and cavorting in wild, ecstatic abandonment.

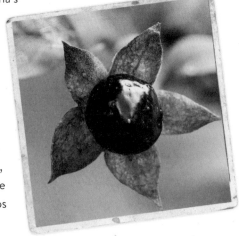

There is a particular Greek myth associated with Atropos, the namesake of the *Atropa belladonna*, that speaks of the formidable nature of this fantastic power plant. Atropos was one of the Moirai, the three Fates who controlled the threads of life and death. The first Fate was Clotho, the spinner. She sits and spins the thread of life, the fabric of human existence. She is the maiden and is often seen in artworks carrying a spindle.

The second Fate was Lachesis, meaning "unbending". She measures out the thread of life which determines how long each person will live. She is the unbending holder of our time spent here in the mortal realm. She is depicted as a matron with a staff with which she points to the horoscope on a globe.

The third Fate is Atropos, meaning "inevitable". She is the cutter of the thread of life, who appears as a crone. She chooses the manner of each person's death and when their time is up; she cuts their life-thread with her shears. Her role is the archetypal death figure. She is the smallest of the three, yet characterized as the most terrible.

The folklore of the three Fates expresses the potential extreme effects of belladonna plant medicine. Of course, it is all in the hands of the person wielding the medicine, as everything is a poison depending on the dose, but as we know some herbs have a narrower therapeutic-to-poisoning dose threshold than others. The common name of "deadly nightshade" is therefore extremely fitting.

BELLADONNA CULTIVATION

Belladonna flowers are like mauve bells with petals that curl back at the entrance to each tiny bell's mouth. And these are the flowers that give way to five green sepals on which its berries sit. The whole plant can grow to up to 5ft (1.5m) tall depending on where it is situated. As we have seen, belladonna is particularly renowned for its jet-black, shiny berries – so enticing and attractive, the berries of temptation. Just observing them and wondering at them is enough ...

To give us more clues about a herb's particular magic and medicine, we love to witness how the seeds of each individual plant germinate. This offers insight into another aspect of their plant traits or personalities. The tiny dark seeds of the belladonna need plenty of patience and perseverance and are definitely the most challenging of our three nightshades to germinate in our experience.

The tiny belladonna seeds, packed with potential, seem to like being soaked for a couple of weeks, with their water changed daily and plenty of attention. A pot of seeds soaking in the water can be placed on your altar space for this time or kept in the fridge.

Then the seeds can be sown in seed trays and kept moist. It can take about two to four weeks before any shoots are visible. Sprinkle over a fine layer of organic potting compost and cover the tray with a lid, cling film or glass to keep the seedlings at a warm temperature and to maintain the moisture. The seedlings should be ready for planting in May, when there is no longer any fear of frost. The plants should be grown 20cm (8in) apart in the first year, with more space required as they grow bigger in the second year.

In the wild, belladonna loves uncultivated or barren areas.

HARVESTING BELLADONNA

You can harvest the different plant parts of the belladonna, and create specific remedies depending on what you want to achieve from her medicine and magic. Once the luscious, dark green leaves have been dried, they can be added into

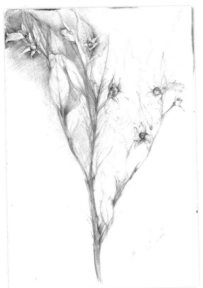

oils in preparation for the flying ointment (see Part III). The roots are thick and fleshy and, once all the soil is washed away, white in colour, and can be dried or made into fresh tinctures for clinical applications.

As the flowers fall away, they reveal those attractive dark berries that create a fabulous dye. You can make vibrant magical inks with this enchanting, vivid purple juice, and draw on this colourful fluid for shadow work and magic.

For seed saving, scrape the minuscule, dot-like seeds away from the flesh of the berry, dry them off and store in paper bags in a cool, dry space.

BELLADONNA IN HEALING

There is a long history of belladonna uses as an external preparation in the form of "medicine-filled gauzes", which were previously applied for a number of different treatments. These include so-called psychiatric disorders, as well as excessive sweating and bronchial asthma. However, as we have seen, over the years many of the Solanaceae alkaloids have fallen out of common use due to their unpredictable side effects and induced delirium with larger doses.

In our work exploring Sensory Herbalism we often give people a single drop of a simple tincture in order for them to experience the intricate tastes, and also the qualities and actions of the herb. People report increased focus after just one drop of the belladonna tincture, expressing heightened sensitivity, feelings of being more alert and increased visual clarity.

Atropa belladonna has been described again and again by the hundreds of participants in our workshops as a medicine that increases awareness and improves focus. It is an upward-moving herb that clears the mind, improves vision and heightens the senses. Belladonna is thought to ready one for intellectual work. It is neither high and giddy, nor introspective and deep. This, of course, doesn't apply to larger doses, but to the subtle energetics of the plant.

EXTERNAL PREPARATIONS OF BELLADONNA

From the middle of the 19th century to the late 1950s, belladonna was incorporated in the external applications of plasters (waxy or oily preparations mixed with herbs and applied with a cloth or gauze to bring heat, reduce inflammation or reduce pain) and liniments (usually in oil form to use as a rub to relieve pain). These preparations were used to treat a wide variety of conditions, including neuralgia, chronic rheumatism, lumbago, myalgia, pleurisy, pulmonary tuberculosis and acute mastitis.

Belladonna-laced preparations like this were purchased over the counter at pharmaceutical chemists and apothecaries. One has to remember that seeing a doctor was expensive; thus these pain-relieving items often saved great expense.

Considerable relief can be obtained in muscular pains and aches by the skilful use of a well-prepared plaster or liniment. We have seen great results with these preparations over the years in our own practice.

ALCOHOLICS ANONYMOUS AND BELLADONNA

American doctors called it the "belladonna cure". It was first developed in Europe by German chemists who extracted hyoscine from the belladonna plant and started to experiment with it in the treatment of morphine addicts (morphine addiction being a huge issue in the early 1900s). The drug was shown to be useful and American doctors worked with it first with people suffering from mania and then with alcoholics and those with other addictions such as to opium or cocaine. However, the belladonna treatment of the 1920s was usually for those less well-off and often a brutal affair. The rich would have had personalized, opulent care, while the poor would have been locked up in awful asylums, suffering from potentially induced delirium – all in the name of a cure!

Nevertheless, there are many US hospital reports of so-called epiphanies, or access to knowledge previously unknown from patients under the influence of psychotropic and mind-altering belladonna compounds. The foundation of the global organization Alcoholics Anonymous was born after one such vision by a man called Bill Wilson. Wilson had met God when under the influence of the "belladonna cure" for his alcoholism. His room was completely filled with light and a cleansing wind blew in; he became freed of his addiction. He went on to set up the 12-step programme that is now a huge movement in the support of overcoming alcohol addiction. We like to think that the fierce grace of this herb played some role in establishing this awesome organization.

In our own work, we have encountered and supported many people suffering with addiction issues, and have found the consciousness-altering and sedative plants to be super useful in treatment strategies. The experience of living on traveller sites and being part of the UK free party scene in the 1990s gave us the opportunity to see how effective herbal medicines can be with tackling alcohol withdrawal symptoms. One of our plants of choice is valerian, which in high doses is incredibly effective in promoting sleep –

something that often evades alcoholics as they attempt to free themselves of their dependence. There can also be intense tremors present. Both these symptoms of sleeplessness and tremors point to the use of Solanaceae herbs, with their anti-spasmodic and sedative actions. Much care is needed around dosage, however, to ensure a threshold isn't crossed, creating a whole new set of issues. Large-dose treatment with hyoscine ceased due to the severe delirium that it can cause.

BELLADONNA EYE MEDICINE

If you or your family and friends have ever had eye problems, investigations or surgery, you may very well have been prescribed ophthalmic atropine, which would have been dropped directly into your eye in order to dilate the pupil. It is also used to relieve pain caused by swelling and inflammation of the eye.

In the form of ophthalmic atropine drops, belladonna is a valued plant in the treatment of eye diseases. The alkaloid atropine, extracted from the plant, is responsible for the plant's pupil-dilating action and has been applied for this action for centuries. Atropine will dilate the pupils whether used internally or dropped directly into the eyes. When applied directly into the eye, a much smaller dose is needed, and fewer systemic effects occur.

During the time of the Renaissance, the ladies of the Venetian court would drop the juice of the belladonna berry into their eyes for the mydriasis (pupil enlargement) it caused, as dilated pupils were considered more alluring.

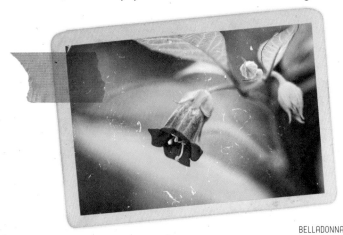

171

Belladonna Eye Drops

Here is a treatment championed by medical herbalist Geoffrey Soma for treating migraine onset. Mix equal amounts of *Atropa belladonna* tincture with water. Then take two drops of this combination in the eye of the worst affected side of the head, three minutes apart, up to three doses or until symptoms subside.

We have applied a similar method to a patient whose migraines managed to reduce from several a month to once monthly but which could still be debilitating when they arose. This was through using a similar dilution in distilled water that was applied as one drop followed by a 10- to 20-minute wait. The dose was repeated as needed and the patient felt that it prevented her migraines from coming on as severely as they had been doing, and stopped them from lasting as long. She continued to use this method for the following couple of months until her migraines became even less frequent.

After using undiluted belladonna tincture directly in the eye, some folk have recounted their vision being affected for up to two weeks afterwards, and also the pupil taking a long time, sometimes days, to return to normal. To avoid using alcohol from the tincture directly into the eye, it has been suggested that juice from the berries diluted in water can be used. The pupil in the eyes will usually constrict to protect the eyes from UV light damage, so it is recommended that people receiving the tincture wear protective sunglasses until their pupils return to normal.

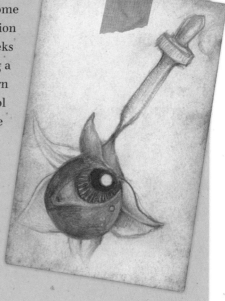

THE ANTISPASMODIC ACTION OF BELLADONNA

In our clinical practice, belladonna has proved invaluable for its antispasmodic action in the treatment of Parkinson's disease, to reduce the severity of the debilitating tremors. Parkinson's disease is a degeneration of dopamine neurones within the basal ganglia. Before the discovery of dopamine-enhancing drugs such as Levodopa, belladonna was the main pharmacological treatment for Parkinson's disease. Belladonna is also prescribed to help relieve the excessive saliva production and drooling that develops in later stages of Parkinson's disease, because of the action of the tropane alkaloids that dry up saliva caused by cholinergic innovation in Parkinson's.

Belladonna is known for its antispasmodic action on the GI tract. Rudolf Fitz Weiss, a well-known German herbalist of the late 20th century, states that belladonna is a superior GI antispasmodic due to its strongest action to relax smooth (involuntary) muscles – the whole herb tincture causes reactions that are more intensive than any chemical drug, as it also has the ability to suppress secretions.

Belladonna is an excellent herb for acute treatments, and can be used where there are any spasmodic pains, severe sweats, violent mood swings or confusion. We have seen the medicine work wonders in acute pain management, helping to alleviate spasms and griping intestinal agonies in just a few moments.

HOT FLUSHES

In our clinical experience, belladonna has always reduced the severity and frequency of hot flushes in patients.

Flushes and sweats can be extremely debilitating, interfering with day-to-day life. In these instances, belladonna can be used to support the symptomatic relief of menopausal sweats while the other factors are addressed over a longer period of time.

When attempting to relive hot flushes with herbal medicine, a holistic approach should be taken by considering all the underlying issues while exploring ideas around adrenal fatigue, stress and digestion.

BELLADONNA AND CLINICAL HERBALISM

Belladonna's use as a medicine has walked alongside humanity from antiquity to the present day, each shift of medical paradigm bringing with it varied approaches to use. To quote Professor Michael Heinrich of UCL School of Pharmacy, when it comes to belladonna:

> The deadly dose can be very low. A berry can kill a small child. It certainly is a classical case of a highly toxic plant, but it all depends on the form of administration, the dose, and other circumstances, the person's characteristics (age, size, preconditions).

Medicinal tinctures of belladonna are made at a 1 in 10 ration of herb to alcohol at 70 per cent proof. The dose is recommended at 2.5 to 10ml per week of tincture for 10 to 14 days, depending on the reason for use.

Belladonna's alkaloids are prescribed today as anticholinergic agents to assist with everything from treating GI issues in patients with Parkinson's to asthma and Chronic Obstructive Pulmonary Disorder (CPOD). Compounds extracted from belladonna are used in modern pharmaceutical medicine as active ingredients in many drugs, including insomnia medications, to decrease saliva production, to counteract bradycardia (slow heart rate) and anti-nausea drugs. Atropine is the major compound extracted from belladonna for use in modern pharmaceutical medicine.

A SOOTHING OINTMENT

Medical herbalist Katherine Bellchambers-Wilson uses belladonna topically to treat acute intervertebral disc prolapse. She uses one part each of Atropa belladonna, Viburnum opulus *and* Lobelia inflata, *to be applied topically. Katherine also uses belladonna as part of a cream for painful joints and muscles.*

You will need:

- ∗ *50g (½ cup) base cream or comfrey cream*
- ∗ *5ml (1 tsp) each of* Atropa belladonna, Gelsemium sempervirens *and* Lobelia inflata *tinctures*
- ∗ *10ml (2 tsp)* Hypericum perforatum *tincture*
- ∗ *10 drops lavender essential oil*
- ∗ *4 drops chamomile blue essential oil*

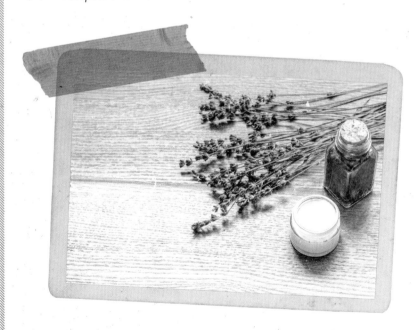

BELLADONNA FLOWER ESSENCE

The flowers of belladonna can be prepared into an essence, summoning an energy of "fierce grace", offering the power of transformation by aiding us to see setbacks as launching pads for a new viewpoint. In this way, the essence potentiates visualization. It empowers us to greet adversity square on, look it in the eye and cut away anything that is holding us back, thus enabling the embrace of raw energy of life present to us in any given moment.

The flower essence offers us the ability to be prepared for challenge and change. The sludge of life that can often bring a feeling of moving through treacle, slowing everything down to almost a halt – which marks the perfect moment to reach for your belladonna bloom essence. This essence gives us second sight, attuning our inner eye to see clearly what needs pruning from our lives and ways in which we can accomplish this efficiently. This can bring the impetus to keep on rolling with the punches, moving forward finding the joy in among the sludge.

BELLADONNA EARTH MAGIC

There are particularly auspicious times for spell-work with belladonna. If creating ceremonial inks with belladonna berries, for example, work at a time when the moon is transiting through one of the Air signs of Aquarius, Gemini and Libra. Belladonna spell-work is greatly enhanced by these astrological signs.

The element of Air blows away negative energies and allows us to tap into imagination and communion with the mercurial forces of intellect and quick wit. This will enhance the power of your ceremonial inks, aiding any and all communications that your writings in these plant and Earth bloods result in.

MAKE YOUR OWN CEREMONIAL INK

Today, much modern ink contains petroleum oils and therefore heavy metals, but we can easily return to a more natural way. When writing down spells, nothing beats working with the ingredients of nature in the form of homemade inks created from fruits, barks, berries and plant roots.

Charcoal stabilizes well but other natural additives can be added to create more longevity for the inks you create. Many natural colours are available – from the deep browns of walnut to the rich deep reds of elderberry. Belladonna's purple devil's cherries make a fairy-tale vibrant ink that is perfect for writing out charms. You can write ritualistic words, specific spells, poems, wishes and incantations with your super-special magical belladonna ink. However, while working with the berries please remember that the juice is potent, so wear gloves!

Belladonna spell-work is greatly enhanced by the astrological Air signs of Aquarius, Gemini and Libra, so for added potency work when the moon is transiting one of these signs.

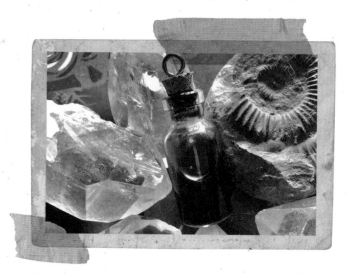

You will need:

* 3–5 leaves foraged from four types of plant, such
  as nettle, plantain, dock or horse chestnut
* 13 belladonna berries
* 200ml (7fl oz) water
* 2 heaped tsp salt
* 3 tbsp white vinegar
* gum arabic (available at art-supply stores)
* 10 drops of whole clove or wintergreen essential oil
* rubber gloves
* an old pot (stainless steel works best)
* coffee filter
* funnel
* wide-mouthed glass jar
* small glass bottle with lid
* labels (optional)

Steps:

1. Put on your rubber gloves and place all your natural ingredients in
   an old pot. Heat the brew, keeping it to just below boiling point.
2. Simmer on a low heat for at least an hour, with a lid on
   to prevent evaporation, or until water takes on a deep,
   rich colour. Use a strip of paper to test the colour.
3. Place a coffee filter inside the funnel, then put
   the funnel inside a wide-mouth glass jar. Pour the
   water slowly into the funnel to filter the ink.
4. In a glass bottle, add gum arabic (1 part to 10 parts ink)
   and 10 drops of whole clove or wintergreen essential oil as a
   preservative. Pour your ink into the bottle, leaving some space
   at the top. Close with a tight-fitting lid and label if you wish.

- 9 -

HOMOEOPATHY AND THE WITCHING HERBS

odern homoeopathy is a controversial subject that is often confused with herbalism. We have been asked if herbalism is homoeopathy countless times and it is perplexing to a lot of people that it isn't one and the same thing – but it is not! They are vastly different practices.

Homoeopathy regularly provokes heated arguments as to whether its theory and practice are valid or just pseudoscience. In fact, homoeopathy is perhaps one of the most misunderstood and hotly debated topics in the field of medicine. For some people, it is their main system of healing and they swear by it. In the UK, many of us will have grown up with the sight of those familiar small pill bottles of the most popular remedies, such as arnica and indeed belladonna, on sale in virtually every high-street chemist and pharmacy. Homoeopathic belladonna is commonly used to treat childhood fevers, allowing many infants have an energetic "hit" of this power plant even before they eat solid foods!

Samuel Hahnemann (1755–1843) is often called the father of homoeopathy. He was a learned doctor from Germany who created his own system of medicine after becoming disappointed with the dominant medicine of his time. Hahnemann believed that the conventional form of medicine he had been taught to practise sometimes did the patient more harm than good and he set about designing a – in his opinion – better way of practising. As a multi-linguist, he found work translating medical and scientific texts, from which he learned about wide-ranging ideas and philosophies, and new and old techniques in healthcare.

THE HOMOEOPATHIC PICTURE

A "homoeopathic picture" is created by carefully profiling an individual patient's personality and habits, which are then studied alongside their physical and emotional symptoms. The resulting picture unlocks important insights into which remedies might be most suitable and is analysed by an experienced practitioner in order to find the correct remedy.

In our own practice, we are particularly interested in research done in relation to the henbane, datura and belladonna homoeopathic remedies and the types of people they have an affinity with and can be used to treat. We have studied many writings on homoeopathic profiling, which has proved very helpful for understanding these three Solanaceae herbs even more deeply.

When working clinically with our own patients and thinking about which of the Solanaceae herbs to reach for in their treatment, the information made available through homoeopathic studies has been extremely useful to reference. While the system is not at all directly transferable to herbalism, it certainly provides useful insights on how to allocate the different plants to different personality profiles. For example, a person might come to us with severe asthma. Datura is the most famous herb of the three for applications in asthma, but the patient might fit a henbane picture a lot more clearly, thus giving us pause for thought and further reflection in our work. The same goes for treating menopausal sweats: belladonna is the most well-established treatment of the three but henbane may be more pertinent to the individual's homoeopathic picture or profile.

To be clear, we do not practise or prescribe homoeopathic remedies, but we find the observations in homoeopathic texts valid and a source of useful information. The way Hahnemann worked with the plants was to sit with them and explore their energetic qualities. This shares much with the way we work with herbs initially.

As previously mentioned, the way we prescribe and apply the power plant herbs is generally in drop doses ranging from one drop to 13 drops depending on the individual and their reasons for taking them. This drop dosing causes many diverse interactions and responses in the physical body, as even in a single drop of herbal tincture there are phytochemicals present. Even though this is a small dose, it most definitely isn't homoeopathy as homoeopathy works with vibrations and not actual chemical compounds.

HOMOEOPATHIC PROFILE FOR HENBANE

Henbane is known as Hyoscyamus or Hyos in homoeopathy.

One peculiar symptom that is subscribed to a Hyoscyamus type is the desire to uncover or to kick the bedclothes off.

The most common symptoms experienced by Hyoscyamus people include a confused state of the mind, agitated behaviour, murmuring or grumbling and indecent or lewd sexual exhibitionism. Hyoscyamus people may also be found to laugh out loud at the wrong times and come across as socially awkward.

Hyoscyamus can be prescribed homoeopathically to treat physical disorders that are associated with uncontrolled trembling. The Hyoscyamus patient can be racked by convulsions, contractions, trembling, quivering and jerking of the muscles. The Hyoscyamus person's movements are unlike the gyratory motions of the Stramonium (datura) type, but include coarse angular jerks that hurl the patient about.

HOMOEOPATHIC PROFILE FOR DATURA

Datura is known as Stramonium in homoeopathy.

The Stramonium patient cannot walk in the dark or with their eyes shut as it makes them unstable to the extreme and they are generally frightened of the darkness.

The spasmodic motions of Stramonium are characterized by gracefulness rather than angularity; they are more gyratory than jerking. The picture of the patient might include sexual obsession or nymphomania.

Stramonium is used in the treatment of fear, anxiety and panic disorders such as PTSD and panic attacks.

HOMOEOPATHIC PROFILE FOR BELLADONNA

Belladonna is known simply as belladonna in homoeopathy.

The face of the belladonna patient is often red and flushed, and their eyes seem to glisten. They are not easily ignored or passed by, but tend to stand out in the crowd.

A belladonna character will grind their teeth and in general those who sleep with them will tell you of the intense activity that characterizes their sleep. They often suffer from hypersensitivity to light, noise and even touch when they are ill. They are also sensitive to quick changes in temperature, and prone to irritability, a history of impatience and sudden flares of temper. They might struggle to control various compulsions to violence – for example, a temptation to bite or pull someone's hair.

Belladonna should also be thought of in conditions like pyromania and kleptomania. Great emphasis is placed on the "suddenness" of belladonna conditions. More than anything, these types are excitable people.

SOME FINAL THOUGHTS ON HOMOEOPATHY

These homoeopathic accounts of our three herbs and diverse character associations offer only a brief overview of an incredible wealth of observations spanning over hundreds of years. These observations tie in with much of our own understanding about the effects of henbane, datura and belladonna when working in subtler emotional and energetic ways. We find it very affirming to have arrived at similar conclusions through our personal experiences and working with groups. It seems that people from centuries apart can ascertain similar information from working energetically with the same herbs. That in itself is magic!

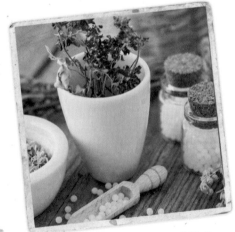

- 10 -
A HEX FOR THE WILD

o book on herbal poisons and power plants could be complete without a reference to curses, more commonly referred to as hexes. We have touched upon this challenging topic briefly in Chapter 2, but now it's time to explore it in more depth. One of the main fears associated with witches is their power to direct their will and create very real consequences, for both healing and malevolence. With these revered power plants, there is similarly the power to kill or cure. So what creates the distinction between a hex cast with ill intent, and one for potential good? What exactly is a curse? And where do they originate?

Archaeologists have found many examples of ancient inscribed curse tablets, which the Greeks called *katares*, "curses that bind tight". These have been discovered in graves, wells and fountains – places where the dead could better work their magic. Tablets were also written for matters of the heart and love spells, but when magic was drawn on for this they were placed inside the home of the desired target, rather than at the site of a potential threshold between worlds.

As discussed earlier, the general understanding within spellcraft is that what you put out there creates a flow of attracting energy that leads back to you. You must be aware and prepared for the fact that where your energy goes, so follows the energy of the Earth.

It nevertheless seems a little too binary to suggest that there are only inherently "good" or inherently "bad" actions. If all magic is the manipulation of energy to bend events to our will, this can work for both selfish and altruistic outcomes. The universal oneness, it would seem, is not programmed to respond only to benevolent requests. The universal flow responds according to our will.

For this reason, we will be working with the idea of casting hexes, or curses, where there is a bigger picture or intended outcome. There needs to be a flow and an understanding of consequences ... one spell or hex does not occur and then stop. There are reverberations of energy bending that occur. This is why we recommend that you work backward: what are the desired outcomes? With these in mind, what is the best choice of intention and how will this be carried out or performed? You can then connect herbs and their energetics to the desired outcomes to add power to the intention.

Your own magical practices will, like ours, be developed over years of exploring and connecting with nature and the esoteric realms. Allow your spellcraft to be led by the plants themselves. Tap into the individual gifts or energetics of the herbs, their folklore and deity associations, and, when a certain situation arises, consider what fits best if you wish to carry out a change or shift to enhance the flow of energy. As you fine-tune your craft, keep in mind your intentions and their possible repercussions for the good or ill of all.

A HEX FOR OUR TIMES

Here in the heart of our book you find a spell, a hex that draws on the individual energetics of *Atropos belladonna* – a hex on wonton consumerism. We would love to see an end to the constant unsustainable growth of capitalism and to an addiction to consumerism driven by fear of lack. The modern world has seen an obsession with the growth economy ... a desire to remain in the constant summer energy of growing bigger, bigger, bigger. This entirely unsustainable attitude has seen the destruction of much of the planet – the decimation of plant life and habitats for animals, along with heightened fluctuations in the weather, and the pollution of the seas and the air we breathe.

People often refer to "them", "those people" and "they" as if there were one entity in control of world decisions and aims. For this hex, we propose that there is no single one governing party that determines the future of society, but rather there is a series of interactions between the natural world, social movements and economic development. With this in mind we can conjecture that because society has changed through the course of a series of key movements and moments in time, it can change again.

Capitalism is referred to as having started with the industrialization of society. There were many steps along the way to this in the UK – from the feudal system of localized control of peasant populations to the rise of the merchant classes and colonization. The system we know today as capitalism began in around the 1700s. Most of these stages were arguably driven by the need for power and control – stemming from a fear of lack. We will therefore be targeting the energetic source of this fear in our hex.

We are calling upon Atropos to hex these energetic fear entities. The great shifts that will occur on the back of this wish will entail great hardship with the necessary adjustments. This is inevitable, so it is key to ask that this be initiated and held with as much grace, compassion and kindness as possible.

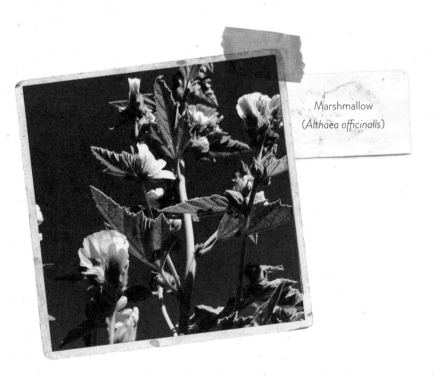

Marshmallow
(*Althaea officinalis*)

A HEX ON WANTON CONSUMERISM

Belladonna seems a fitting herb to hold a hex to end the capitalist society as we know it, and to move into a new phase or era. Held by belladonna, and with henbane, datura, mandrake, rose and marshmallow, we initiate a hex that is important to us, adding fuel to our life's work.

Marshmallow is the archetypical traditional nurse; steadfast and caring, she never seems to tire, is always present and in support and service. The Latin name for marshmallow, Althaea officinalis, comes from Althea the goddess of healing. It is extremely important in this work to recognize that in place of the thing that you are banishing, there needs to be care, support and love to fill the gap.

Rose not only represents secrecy but also protection and love. She invites the tribe to gather under her petals and form strong bonds of love to walk toward the dream of a more positive, wholesome future.

Mandrake is included in this spell as a symbol and source of fertility on Earth, to allow the new vision to grow, powerful and connected.

This curse is greatly enhanced by working when the dark moon is transiting one of the Earth signs of Taurus, Virgo and Capricorn. We are using the power of the Earth energy to ground this hex and bring it back to the Earth, whom we choose to nourish, restore and replenish with our devotion and love.

The intention of this hex is to bring the death or ending to profit-focused consumeristic capitalism, with a focus on encouraging vitality, nourishment and diversity back into the natural world. It is important to note that we don't ask blindly of the consequences. We call for all beings to be free of suffering, and for peace and harmony on our planet.

You will need:

* 2 naturally dyed dark candles
* 1 cup marshmallow tea
* 1 tsp datura seeds
* 1 tsp henbane seeds
* 1 tsp belladonna seeds
* 1 tsp rose petals
* piece of mandrake root
* 1 dagger
* 1 pair scissors
* length of dark ribbon
* length of string
* notebook and pen
* rose cream or oil

Steps:

1. Light the candles in order to provide protective fire energy for your safe space, and put them in secure holders on your altar, keeping the flames away from drafts and flammable fabrics.
2. Cast your circle for protection.
3. Sit in front of your altar with all your tools to hand. Take a moment to relax and steady your thoughts. Take a sip of your tea and focus on the supportive healing powers of marshmallow.
4. Sprinkle the seeds and rose petals on your altar and place the mandrake root there too.
5. Now pick up the dagger and repeat:

   Over the din of humanity

   Hear my appeal!

   Let materialism

   Decrease, diminish, drop,

   Die!

6. Put the dagger on the altar, pick up the scissors and ribbon. Repeat:

I call upon Atropos,
Sister of Clotho and Lachesis,
I evoke your energy of finality,
I evoke the power of your scissors –
Cut all ties to fears,
Fears of lack ...

7. Cut the ribbon, then place it on the altar with the scissors. Repeat:

I call on you, Henbane –
Take us all on a journey
Across rivers where
Capitalism and Greed are no more.

I call on you, Datura –
Shift and shape this future time
With moon-bathed beauty.

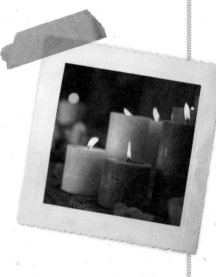

I call on you, Belladonna –
Enable a new vision
Open all eyes to
Nature's abundance.

I call on you, Rose,
To hold all of life with
Protection, Harmony and
Peace.

8. Sit quietly and allow these words to rise into the Universe.
9. Now pick up the length of string. This is going to represent a nature-focused, interactive utopia whereby nature is seen by all as something that we love and connect with. The Earth becomes a place where we are custodians rather than masters of the land around us; a place where nature is part of our playground that we tend and care for, rather than somewhere we destroy or view as wallpaper, there only for our own entertainment.
10. Now visualize plants, trees, birds, insects, animals, humans – all existing together. A world of peace, cooperation, care and diversity.
11. Lay the string out in front of you and visualize the start of it as a land where people are part of nature. They respond to the environment and are governed by nature as much as they govern it. The plant world interacts with humans, with the plant world using humans for seed dispersal, and in turn providing medicine, clothing and shelter.
12. Rub a little rose cream or oil into the area over your heart space and take three long, deep breaths.
13. Brainstorm a list of services or gifts that you could offer within your local environment. This can be anything, but here are some ideas to get you started:

* A local litter-pick.
* Noting down the herbs that grow in a local area and producing an information sheet for local people to access.
* Observing the local environment and noticing changes that could make a difference to the plants and animals in your area. Petition the relevant agencies for support, finance or information.
* Join a local group – Friends of… (your local woods, park, coastline) – and offer time or support for their work.
* Organize information days in your local area, like a herb walk or a fungi foray, or join days that are already happening to

become acquainted with the natural world around you.

* Create a map of all the tree species in your local area
  and make a map or trail for local people to follow.
* Create seed bombs of native seeds that fit in
  with the local environment and guerrilla garden
  where diversity is lacking (see page 191).
* Find out about the water quality and diversity of life in your
  local river and what is being done to support or aid this.

14. Choose a couple of the ideas that you can realistically carry out.
    Write them out separately in your notebook and commit to them.
15. As you tie a knot in the string for each one of your ideas,
    repeat out loud three times (once for yourself, once for the
    natural world and once for the Universe to hear you):

    I make a promise to the natural world to [your chosen action].

16. When you are ready, end this ritual reverently
    and close your sacred space.
17. In the weeks that follow, carry your string with you, tied with knots,
    as a reminder of the pledge you've made to the natural world.

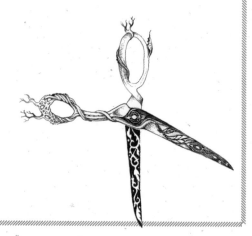

MAKE YOUR OWN SEED BOMBS

Seed bombs are a brilliant and fun way to bring some life to any hard-to-reach or barren areas. These ones are made with the henbane, datura, belladonna and marshmallow seeds and can be charged with your intentions to create change.

You will need:

* mixing bowl
* seeds of marshmallow, henbane, datura, belladonna
* organic peat-free compost
* clay soil or powdered clay
* water

Steps:

1. In a bowl, mix together 1 cup of seeds with 5 cups of compost and 23 cups of clay soil or powdered clay.
2. Slowly mix in water with your hands until everything sticks together.
3. Roll the mixture into firm balls and leave to dry in a sunny spot.
4. Plant your seed bombs by throwing them at barren ground – as long as they are watered they will grow.

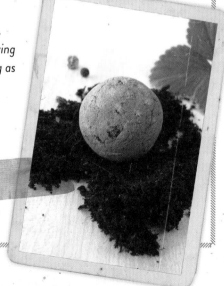

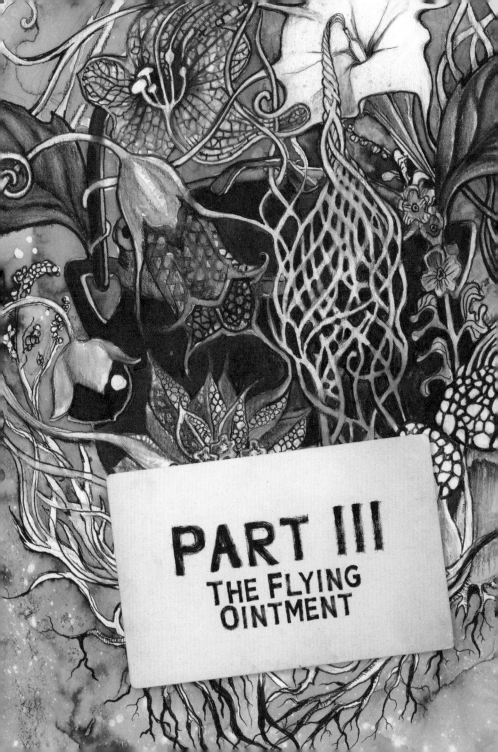

PART III
THE FLYING OINTMENT

"EVERYONE DESERVES A CHANCE TO FLY."

ELPHABA, *WICKED*

The flying ointment is a magical mythological preparation that has captured the imagination of many throughout the ages. It is potentially the missing link to the safe therapeutic use of the Solanaceae plants for healing on many levels. Most reports on the recreational use of the Solanaceae plants date from Western culture in the 1970s and, as we have seen earlier in this book, describe the ingestion of simple infusions or use by smoking. However, none of them reflect the apparent ethnobotanical sophistication of the green ointment. In this part we will explore the history of this preparation and how we can interpret it today. We will share our own flying ointment recipe and considering therapeutic applications for the ointment, as well as how we can use it alongside another potent brew – the Passion Potion.

– 11 –

THE HISTORY OF THE
FLYING OINTMENT

reen ointment, witch's balm, hallucinogenic lube, *unguentum sabbati* ... the flying ointment is known by many names, but first and foremost is famed for its use as a psychotropic preparation by European medieval and modern witches.

This Solanaceae-rich ointment was probably applied to the mucous membranes of the vagina with a smooth broomstick handle or other handily shaped implement. Its effects create a sense of flying high; hence it became a part of the folklore of witches flying on their broomsticks. Stories were once rife of wanton women flying with their witch sisters at the Sabbats to wild woodland meets at turning points of the year. Pious medieval Christians such as the writer of the 13th-century *A Diatribe against Witches* believed that these horny happenings must have been "obvious devilish or hellish involvement".

Springing from the Celtic tradition, the pagan celebrations known as the Sabbats are Samhain, Yule, Imbolc, Ostara, Beltane, Litha, Lughnasadh and Mabon. The dates for those Sabbats linked to the solstices and equinoxes vary slightly from year to year because our Gregorian calendar system does not match the reality of the Earth's orbit around the sun.

As we have seen, magic practices throughout history have been influenced by people's local plants, landscapes and people. The Solanaceae plants of Britain provide powerful physical medicines but also alter the state of consciousness. When we work with magically ritualized herbs in the flying ointment, it is clear that they have gifts to offer far beyond those of physical pain relief.

The Sabbats and their Dates

DATE	ENGLISH NAME	CELTIC NAME
31 October	Halloween (All Hallows' Eve)	Samhain
19–22 December	Winter Solstice	Yule
1 February	Candlemas	Imbolc
19–22nd March	Spring Equinox	Ostara
1 May	May Day	Beltane
19–22 June	Summer Solstice	Litha
1 August	Harvest Festival	Lughnasadh
19–22 September	Autumn Equinox	Mabon

These Sabbats were and are times associated with merriment
and rituals – and application of the flying ointment.

As we have explored previously, the Solanaceae can produce similar experiences among all its users, regardless of a person's belief system or intention. Common reports under intoxication with the Solanaceae include accounts of creatures crawling all over the body, visions of hair-covered figures, losing time (hours passing but seeming like minutes) and hallucinations that appear real.

These phenomena have been documented since the mid-1500s when Andrés Laguna, who served as a physician to the Spanish King, started to look more deeply into the effects of plants that were being confiscated during the witch trials. Laguna was a scholar and medicine researcher. He set about trying to prove that the visions folk were having came directly from the plants themselves, and not from direct communion with the Devil. He even showed that the wife of a local executioner, a God-fearing woman, had undergone similar experiences as those who were deemed witches. His work was swiftly shut down on pain of death.

An atmosphere of forced belief in the occult and devil worship ensured the suppression of the medicine women and their knowledge. If there was no belief in satanic worship, then the argument that the so-called "witches" were dangerous fell apart. It is perhaps no surprise that all sorts of claims were made about the nature of the flying ointment itself, including Reginald Scot's description in *The Discoverie of Witchcraft*, published in 1584:

> [take]... the fat of yoong children, and seeth it with water in a brasen vessell, reserving the thickest of that which remaineth boiled in the bottome, which they laie up and keep, until occasion serveth to use it. They put hereunto eleoselinum, aconitum, frondes populeas, and soote.

From this text you can see how fear and lies about witches were spread. The true nature of the ointment was rather less horrific, though still extraordinary.

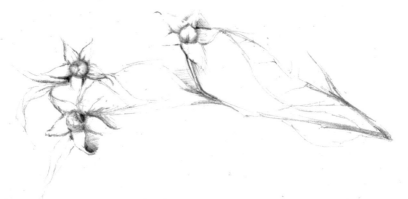

THE ORIGINS OF THE FLYING OINTMENT

The flying ointment is traditionally a green unguent, or fat- or oil-based balm. It is full of psychotropic plants and fungi in combination with other herbal allies that potentiate and protect. The alkaloid-rich fat or oil that forms the traditional base of a flying ointment is generally coloured green from the plant material itself; hence another of the ointment's names: "the green ointment".

Traditionally, animal fats were used to extract the potent oils and alkaloids from these powerful plants as they were convenient and accessible, even to the poor. Today, with the help of modern science, we know that our skin will absorb a salve made with pig's lard more quickly and easily than any other substance because our genetics are so similar. However, in our flying ointment recipe we prefer to use almond or olive oil.

As we've seen, the Solanaceae plant family has been used across the globe both for reaching altered states and as physical medicine. However, we may never completely know how and why these psychoactive plants were first utilized in the flying ointment. In the same way, knowledge about the extent of the ointment's use for ritual and magic remains misty.

It is often held that us of the witches' flying ointment only dates back to the Early Modern era, as the majority of written accounts and recipes are from that period. But there are myths and pre-Christian lore that describe fat-based ointments that bestowed powers of flight. The oldest reference is from Homer's *Iliad* (c. 800 BCE), in which the goddess Hera uses an oil of ambrosia to fly to Olympus, never touching the Earth.

The witching herbs are steeped in a tumultuous past and bring with them powerful archetypes. They are representative of the witch, the midwife, the healer, and symbolize personal responsibility, freedom, wisdom and knowledge.

Recipes for flying ointments were spoken of in hushed tones down through the generations, from grandmother to daughter, those called sorcerer or witch, those keepers of the secret knowledge.

THE IMPACT OF THE WITCH TRIALS

We have already touched upon the impact of the persecution of witches earlier in this book (see Chapter 2). The witch trials should be seen in the context of new scientific discoveries, increased cultural sophistication and a rise in male-dominated power.

We have to look at what factors made the demonization of women and some male healers possible. It's suggested that one issue was the so-called "mini Ice Age" that occurred during the Middle Ages, when temperatures dropped, winters were prolonged, with large bodies of water freezing over, and the growing season was shortened considerably. These harsh conditions led to crops failing, and people starved and the population declined. A scapegoat was needed.

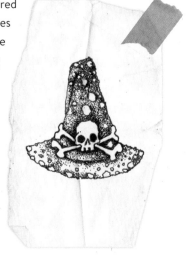

The trials amounted to a genocide of the bearers of traditional, sacred knowledge, and we are still suffering from that loss today. The green ointment was a remedy for muscular spasm and pain, among other applications, yet being found to have this beneficial treatment in your possession at the time of the trials might have sent you to your death.

In England, this period of intense persecution began in 1562 with the Elizabethan Witchcraft Act, which like its 1542 predecessor argued that the practice of magic was real and punishable – sometimes with death.

The Witchcraft Act of 1735 made it a crime to claim that any human being was guilty of practising witchcraft. This later act may have initiated the end of witch trials but it was also influential in pushing magic deep into the underground of a society where even talk of its existence became a crime.

Yet magic cannot be contained forever; like the flow of water, it will always find a way.

- 12 -

THE MAGICAL INGREDIENTS
OF THE FLYING OINTMENT

 hether you believe in serendipity, coincidence or fate, it seems that the native power plants hear your call. Once you begin to work with them, they will start to appear in your tracks.

Our research led us to flying ointment recipes alluded to during the witch trials that included various components such as blood, fat and soot. After many years of researching the plants, we happened to meet 80-year-old Mary walking down a hedged, herbaceous lane in Kernow (Cornwall). She recounted stories of her youth: of sucking foxglove flowers for their nectar on the way home from school and smoking "muggers" (mugwort) wrapped up in paper. It was the start of a wonderful friendship, during which she gifted us with an old herbal, in which we found a handwritten recipe for "the unguent". To our surprise, there listed among other herbs were members of the Solanaceae, as well as soot scraped from the inside of a fire door. This handwritten yellowed paper became the foundation for our flying ointment preparation.

REFINING THE FLYING OINTMENT

After much experimentation and a few adjustments, we settled on our final flying ointment recipe. We bring to this years of study and experience with the Solanaceae family, various fungi, and many other plant friends. There were some traditional ingredients that we decided to include, including soot, and others that we decided to omit, for reasons that will become clear.

THE BENEFITS OF ADDING SOOT

It is debatable whether some of the magical herbal-based practices of the medieval era were recreational, magical or designed for some well-considered medical purpose. In refining our recipe, we researched suggested additives such as soot and the reasons why this might be added to the flying ointment.

Two Italian researchers, Piomelli and Pollio, suggest that at least the inclusion of some excipients (e.g. soot) in Renaissance vegetal ointments probably had a pharmacological rationale. It has been observed that on topical application, tropane alkaloids are slowly absorbed through the skin and that their absorption is enhanced by inducing inflammation, creating abrasions or by using a substance to create an alkaline environment. It seems that the addition of soot to the ointment produced additional alkalinity that would be beneficial for its diffusion into the bloodstream. The effects of applying the ointment topically are much more fast-acting than ingesting the herbs orally.

Piomelli and Pollio suggest that soot's alkalinity could have also changed the profile of some of the more harmful toxic constituents by, for example, turning the alkaloid toxin aconitine into the less harmful derivative aconine. The addition of soot could reduce the potential toxicity of the salve.

During the course of our research, we spoke to toxicologists about the benefits of adding soot, and also of applying the ointment to the mucous membranes, such as vaginally with a broomstick. The rationale behind this is that by applying the ointment directly to the pelvic mucous membranes, the blood that picks up the ointment doesn't go straight to the liver for processing, like it would if the compound was absorbed through the gut. By avoiding being processed in the liver initially, a stronger, more immediate effect can be gained from a smaller amount of the compounds. This could indicate that the ointment has a more powerful, and at the same time potentially less "toxic" effect on the system than oral ingestion of the herbs.

Today, when preparing our flying ointment, we collect soot from various places, such as our log burner or the famous Wookey Hole caves. We always add it to the ointment.

HERBS WE DON'T INCLUDE IN THE OINTMENT

Some of the writings on medieval flying ointment recipes suggest herbs that we have either never worked with, or that we have tried and decided against. After consideration and some experimentation, we have stopped working with two of the herbs altogether: foxglove and hemlock. We don't use these two herbs in any of our flying ointments as we feel that their potential risks are too high. This decision comes as the direct result of our personal experiences with these commonly growing, abundant and commanding plants.

FOXGLOVE

When we studied and connected with the glorious foxglove after our meeting with Mary in Kernow, we discovered this herb to be almost a panacea. We felt the foxglove's effect on our lungs, hearts and kidneys, and also an emotional level – gifting energetic medicine for when there is body dysmorphia. We had some amazing personal experiences with the foxglove, but know this: it is not one for mass consumption, as cumulative toxicity of the foxglove's alkaloids, the cardiac glycosides, can impact negatively on the heart and bring dangers.

Foxglove
(Digitalis purpurea)

Foxglove is, in Britain, one of the herbs used only for pharmaceutical purposes. Medical herbalists are discouraged from working with foxglove as it is under-studied and little is understood about it in clinical herbal practice.

The commonly prescribed heart medication digoxin is extracted from foxglove. After administration of digoxin, a patient's pulse is always taken to carefully monitor their reaction to this powerful medication.

"Mother Hutton", a folk herbalist reputed to live in Shropshire, was said to use foxglove as part of a recipe for dropsy. Dropsy was a term used for the accumulation of fluid in tissues, such as the oedema often caused by congestive heart failure. Botanist and physician William Withering observed Hutton's success at curing dropsy and deduced it was the foxglove that had the clinical effect. Eventually foxglove, which had presumably been commonly used in folk medicine, became restricted in use to pharmacists only, and this has led to a lack of knowledge about the safe use of the herb.

HEMLOCK

There are two poisonous plants with the name hemlock, both in the Apiaceae or Umbellifer family, but each containing different alkaloidal toxic compounds.

Hemlock water dropwort (*Oenanthe crocata*), as the name suggests, is usually found growing in the water. Its toxin acts by constricting or paralysing the muscles, causing death by asphyxia. This effect is also said to be the root of the so-called sardonic grin, evident when prisoners in Phoenician Sardinia were given hemlock water dropwort to end their life. Hemlock water dropwort is considered the most poisonous plant in Britain. All parts of it are poisonous and death can occur as quickly as a couple of hours after ingestion.

Hemlock (*Conium maculatum*) has a purple spotted stem, which gives rise to its Latin name *maculatum*, meaning "with spots".

This hemlock also likes damp conditions and can be found growing mostly in water, although it can grow away from water too. It can grow to be huge in size. Most famed for being the poison that killed Socrates in 399 BCE, as reported by Plato, the toxin in hemlock comes from the compound coniine, which inhibits the central nervous system (CNS), paralysing to the point of respiratory collapse. It would take an estimated six to eight poison hemlock leaves to kill a grown person, but the roots and seeds can be even more potent.

Because of a particularly "closed" and severe vibe we received from these formidable plants, we decided against working with hemlock. We have therefore, never added any part of the herbs to our flying ointment.

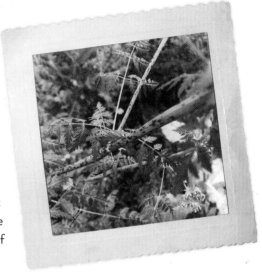

13 HERBS FOR 13 MOONS

Over the years, our recipes have morphed according to where we have travelled, whom we've met and which plants have called to us. These factors also determine which plants are included in our annual ritual of creating the flying ointment, and we have learned a great deal about different blends. This experimental, adaptable way of working has led to many preparations with varying effects. It has also given us an understanding of the most "balanced" combination for our preferred experience, personal tastes and intentions.

Compounds within the herbs act on the body in different ways in accordance with differing preparations. There are differences in which compounds are water-, alcohol- and oil-soluble, for example, and further differences depending on whether they are taken by mouth or applied to mucous membranes externally. Our ancestors might well have prepared these potent toxins in a different way, and they almost definitely would have had completely different relationships with these plants than most of us do today.

As trained herbalists we understand the plant's biochemistry and a little of the intricate dance of each of these compounds and how they interact with

THE MAGICAL INGREDIENTS OF THE FLYING OINTMENT

our human physiology. But there is also the unexplainable power of synergy, with the sum of the distinct compounds being greater when brought together than each of the component parts.

Nature is super-intelligent, always learning and adapting, forever surprising us with her infinite capacity to survive and thrive. As well as the Solanaceae herbs in the flying ointment, we host a supportive cast of integral herbs. Each individual plant invited to the party has a crucial role within the mix. (For some of the plants' astrological associations, please see the table on pages 205–7.)

As you may have gathered by now, the stars of the flying ointment are the henbane, datura and belladonna, bringing all of the gifts we've been illuminating over the pages of this work. However, they shine more brightly if they are joined by some complementary and powerful herbs in their own right to create our famous flying ointment.

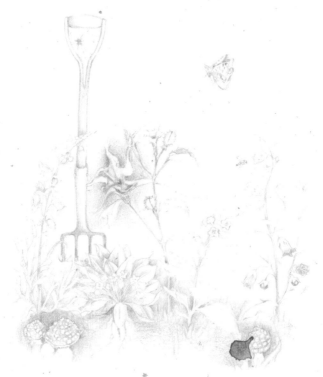

The 13 Herbs of the Flying Ointment

Henbane
FOLK NAMES AND ROLE Apollo's bean (star)
LATIN NAME *Hyoscyamus niger*
INTENTIONS IN RECIPE Celebration of destruction and death, libation
PLANT PARTS USED Aerial parts
LUNAR SIGN OPTIMUM FOR HARVESTING Sagittarius

Datura
FOLK NAMES AND ROLE Moonflower, thorn apple (star)
LATIN NAME *Datura stramonium*
INTENTIONS IN RECIPE Shapeshifting
PLANT PARTS USED Green seed heads
LUNAR SIGN OPTIMUM FOR HARVESTING Scorpio

Belladonna
FOLK NAMES AND ROLE Devil's cherries, deadly nightshade (star)
LATIN NAME *Atropa belladonna*
INTENTIONS IN RECIPE Cutting away of the old
PLANT PARTS USED Aerial parts
LUNAR SIGN OPTIMUM FOR HARVESTING Aries

Aconite
FOLK NAMES AND ROLE Wolfsbane, monkshood (harmony)
LATIN NAME *Aconitum napellus*
INTENTIONS IN RECIPE Flight/astral projection
PLANT PARTS USED Aerial parts
LUNAR SIGN OPTIMUM FOR HARVESTING Aquarius

Mandrake

FOLK NAMES AND ROLE Satan's apple, love apple (harmony)

LATIN NAME *Mandragora officinarum*

INTENTIONS IN RECIPE Fertility

PLANT PARTS USED Root

LUNAR SIGN OPTIMUM FOR HARVESTING Taurus

Mugwort

FOLK NAMES AND ROLE Sailor's tobacco, gypsy's tobacco (harmony)

LATIN NAME *Artemisia vulgaris*

INTENTIONS IN RECIPE Dare to dream

PLANT PARTS USED Flowering aerial parts

LUNAR SIGN OPTIMUM FOR HARVESTING Pisces

Fly agaric

FOLK NAMES AND ROLE Fly agaric (harmony)

LATIN NAME *Amanita muscaria*

INTENTIONS IN RECIPE Storytelling

PLANT PARTS USED Fruiting body

LUNAR SIGN OPTIMUM FOR HARVESTING Pisces

Marshmallow

FOLK NAMES AND ROLE Mortification root, sweet weed (chorus)

LATIN NAME *Althaea officinalis*

INTENTIONS IN RECIPE Invoking healing

PLANT PARTS USED Flowering aerial parts

LUNAR SIGN OPTIMUM FOR HARVESTING Cancer

Yarrow

FOLK NAMES AND ROLE Nosebleed (chorus)

LATIN NAME *Achillea mellifolium*

INTENTIONS IN RECIPE Protection

PLANT PARTS USED Aerial parts
LUNAR SIGN OPTIMUM FOR HARVESTING Gemini

Dandelion
FOLK NAMES AND ROLE Piss-in-bed, clockflower (chorus)
LATIN NAME *Taraxacum officinale*
INTENTIONS IN RECIPE Grounding – keeping a thread to this world
PLANT PARTS USED Root
LUNAR SIGN OPTIMUM FOR HARVESTING Virgo and Capricorn

Fennel
FOLK NAMES AND ROLE Fenkel (chorus)
LATIN NAME *Foeniculum vulgare*
INTENTIONS IN RECIPE Balance and clear communication
PLANT PARTS USED Seeds
LUNAR SIGN OPTIMUM FOR HARVESTING Gemini

Hypericum
FOLK NAMES AND ROLE St John's wort (chorus)
LATIN NAME *Hypericum perforatum*
INTENTIONS IN RECIPE Raising up solar energy
PLANT PARTS USED Aerial parts
LUNAR SIGN OPTIMUM FOR HARVESTING Leo

Rose
FOLK NAMES AND ROLE Damask rose, Turkish rose (chorus)
LATIN NAME *Rosa damascena*
INTENTIONS IN RECIPE Heart-centred love
PLANT PARTS USED Petals
LUNAR SIGN OPTIMUM FOR HARVESTING Libra

THE HARMONIES

To support the stars of the show – henbane, datura and belladonna – in our ointment, we have welcomed in the "harmonies" – aconite, mandrake, mugwort and fly agaric. These plants and fungi potentiate and encourage the psychotropic effects of our three stars. They bring their own gifts to the show – in particular, gifts of intoxication, bringing additional wings. The first of the "harmonies" is the utterly stunning Queen Aconite.

ACONITE/MONKSHOOD

Latin name
Aconite napellus (*napellus* means "little turnip", indicating the shape of its root)

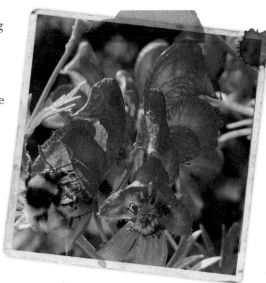

Common names
Aconite, monkshood, wolfsbane

Plant family
Ranunculaceae/buttercup

Astrological ruler
Saturn

Vibe
Flight astral projection

MEDICINE

This purple-hooded beauty is a potent analgesic when used externally. Aconite acts as an anaesthetic for a variety of neurological-related pains, including trigeminal neuralgia, sciatica and joint-related pain such as in lumbago, arthritis, gout and rheumatism.

Aconite initially stimulates and then paralyses nerves that communicate pain, touch and temperature, producing anaesthesia mediated by numerous different alkaloids. The chief toxin alkaloid in the herb is called aconitine and acts by disrupting the normal ion balance in heart-muscle cells. This can cause potentially fatal arrhythmias, including ventricular tachycardia (excessively rapid heart rate), which is the principal cause of death is poisoning cases. Aconite is not recommended for internal use.

In homoeopathic form, "aconite" is used to treat fear, anxiety and restlessness; acute sudden fever; symptoms from exposure to dry, cold weather or very hot weather; tingling, coldness and numbness; influenza or colds with congestion; and heavy, pulsating headaches.

REASON FOR INCLUSION

We once had the pleasure of helping to set up a herb and food garden in a local primary school in which the kids could learn about cultivation. One of the parents, a keen gardener, volunteered on the project with us. We had to laugh when she brought along a few monkshood plants to be planted in the garden. Some gardening books and texts recommend the wearing of gloves while working with this potentially fatal flower. After a short discussion, it was decided they were probably safer in our own garden rather than in the school's! We promptly planted the beautiful perennials in our south-facing front garden where the plants have thrived for the past two decades. The gloriously beautiful blooms and lush foliage of the aconite greet us in the summer months with whispers of magical travel and flight – which is what they offer us in the ointment.

FOLKLORE

This deadly darling is known as the "queen of poisons" in reference to arsenic, known as the "king of poisons". The most poisonous herb in Europe, aconite has a long, murderous history. In the first century CE, the Roman author Pliny reports that the Roman tribune Calpurnius Bestia was accused of killing his wives in their sleep by touching their genitalia with his finger which was smeared with aconite root extracts.

THE MAGICAL INGREDIENTS OF THE FLYING OINTMENT

Aconite is considered one of the earliest herbs to be used as a deadly poison and is mentioned in ancient Greek literature, where it is described as an arrow poison. The Greek word *akónitos* is composed of *ak*, meaning "pointed", and *kônos*, meaning "cone". An *akon* is also a dart or javelin, which is perhaps a reference to the plant's use on arrowheads as well as the shafts, so that an enemy who drew the arrow from the body of a wounded comrade would be poisoned too. Many centuries later, in World War I, modern weapons developers created bullets laced with extracted alkaloids from the herb.

Pliny the Elder recounts that the herb takes its name from Aconae on the Black Sea, the plant's supposed place of origin. Aconae is the spot where Hercules dragged Cerberus, the three-headed hell hound who guarded Hades the underworld. As Cerberus drooled during the fight, poison fell on the plant aconite that grew there, tainting it and making it poisonous forever.

When poisoning occurs, the first effects are like that of a stimulant. Then the toxins soon paralyse the nervous system, causing drooling and vomiting. Finally, the limbs go numb and results in death. The symptom of excessive salivation may be the reason the poison was associated with Cerberus, the hound's foaming drool being poisonous.

There is a white or yellow-flowered species of the plant called *Aconitum lycoctonum*. The plant's Latin name here points to one of the common names by which it is known – wolfsbane. Legend goes that this herb was used to poison wolves by cutting it up in meat left out for them.

The blue flowering aconite that we grow in our own garden is known as monkshood, *Aconitum napellus*. This was once found in medieval monastery gardens. Despite its highly toxic and potentially lethal nature, aconite in the correct dose and formulation was prescribed for a range of different conditions including the relief of stomach spasms.

The two species contain slightly different alkaloid poisons, both of which are lethal.

In India, aconite is sacred to the god Shiva the destroyer, who is, among others, also worshipped as a god of poisons. According to legend, the essence of all poisons (*Hala hala*) spread from the whirling motion of the Ocean of

Milk, Samudramathana, when it produced Kamadhenu, the cow of plenty. The gods were frightened and ran to Mount Kailash, where Shiva sat meditating, and asked him for help. Shiva took the poison in his hands and drank it. His wife Parvati feared for her husband and choked his throat so that the poison would eventually get stuck, upon which his throat turned blue. Because of this Shiva is also called Nilakantha, Blue Throat. Through his deed Shiva saved all beings from becoming poisoned. Only a tiny bit of the poison had dripped from his hand which flows to this day in the veins of the blue aconite and other poisonous plants.

MANDRAKE

Latin name
Mandragora officinarum/autumnalis

Common names
Mandrake, devil's apple, love apple, *Baid-ul-Jinn* (Arabic for "the eggs of the genii")

Family
Solanaceae/nightshade

Astrological ruler
Saturn

Vibe
Fertility

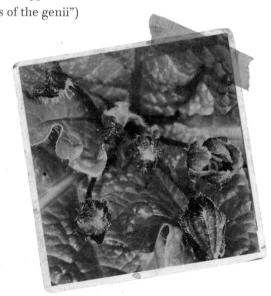

MEDICINE

The second of the harmonies is the mythical mandrake. Like our stars of the show, especially henbane, mandrake has been used as a surgical anaesthetic. Mandrake is part of the medieval recipe for a soporific sponge. Hippocrates, famed as being the Father of Medicine, asserted around 400 BCE that "a small dose in wine, less than would occasion delirium, will relieve the deepest depression and anxiety". Theophrastus, who wrote the first Greek treatise on plants in or around 230 BCE, recommended mandrake as a "sovereign remedy" for sleeplessness.

REASON FOR INCLUSION

We love mandrake, and have been cultivating this perennial companion for many years. We were first given one by a northern witch and we took our new potted friend away with us on a countrywide tour, in pride of place in our travelling apothecary garden. One day, we found ourselves in the Forest of Dean on the border of Wales. We were at an event where the local sheep managed to get in among the stands at the show. They proceeded to graze on the mandrake leaves! We were mortified – had a few moments of not liking sheep – and then wondered how the sheep were. To be honest, they seemed exactly the same as before, although it is quite difficult to read a sheep's mind!

The deep-rooted mandrake is a total wonder plant, full of vital energy. Their resilience is almost unparalleled. Once, having dug up a mandrake root from which to make medicine, we cut away half the root, leaving enough root for the plant to continue growing. The harvested roots were then washed and laid out by the fireplace to dry. Three months later, the drying roots began to sprout new leaves. What an astonishing will to live, lying there dried out – no water, no sunlight, no soil – and still pushing life force through. We re-potted these beauties and they produced healthy, strong plants.

There is something in this story about tenacity, survival and having all the elements needed for growth held in the root even after being uprooted. No outside stimulus was needed for them to thrive against all odds. This plant brings wishes of fertility, prosperity and longevity to the flying ointment.

FOLKLORE

The folklore and historical accounts of the intriguing mandrake are quite bizarre. Seemingly since the dawn of time mandrake has been woven into many a magical spell, used in the summoning of genies and the banishment of demons. Dreams have been written about the herb's connection with fertility. The infamous plant has been regarded with dread, aversion, attraction and allure.

The word "mandrake" may derive from the Old English or Dutch *man drage*. The root looks like the human form, or man, while "drake" is derived from "dragon", referring to the plant's magical powers.

The Greeks associated the plant with two important mythological figures: Circe and Aphrodite. Circe allegedly attempted to bewitch Odysseus with the mandrake but he had taken a preventive antidote (which could have been the snowdrop, *Galanthus*). Furthermore, Aphrodite, goddess of love, was sometimes known as Mandragoritis, or "She of the Mandrake".

One of the earliest writings on mandrake's association with fertility rites can be found in the Old Testament, Genesis, chapter 30, where the childless Rachel asks her sister Leah for the loan of the mandrakes that her son had brought in from the fields. Many a childless couple took to sleeping with a mandrake root under their beds at night, trusting this charm to hold reproductive power.

However, as well as fertility, mandrake was strongly linked to death. The German herbalist Schmidel, writing in 1751, described how mandrake was reputed to grow at the spot where somebody had been executed:

> At the foot of the gallows on which a man has been hanged and where urine has been voided at the time of death, there springs up a plant with broad leaves and a yellow flower. The root of the plant exactly represents the human form, from the hair of his head to the sexual organs.

Mandrake plants generally take about two years to mature, bloom and produce berries and the root can be harvested after three to four years.

Mandrake as Muse

This unusual magical plant has long inspired writers and artists, including the English poet John Donne (1572–1631), who wrote a strange piece called "Song", which included the following verse:

Go and catch a falling star,

   Get with child a mandrake root,

Tell me where all past years are,

   Or who cleft the devil's foot,

Teach me to hear mermaids singing,

Or to keep off envy's stinging,

   And find

   What wind

Serves to advance an honest mind.

MUGWORT

Latin name
Artemisia vulgaris

Common names
Mugwort, gypsy's tobacco,
sailor's tobacco, traveller's
smoke, felon herb

Family
Compositae/daisy

Astrological ruler
Venus

Vibe
Dare to dream

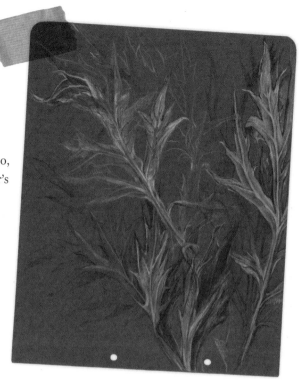

MEDICINE

Mugwort is a bitter tonic; a fantastic digestive herb that creates shifts in stagnant conditions. The herb also has strong nervine action. It affects the perceptions, gently altering the state of consciousness. Working as a uterine stimulant, this plant is an emmenagogue (a substance that increases menstrual flow) and also has diuretic and diaphoretic properties. Its gentle hormone-balancing effects aid a graceful acceptance of "what is". Sometimes not being able to function and being completely vulnerable are exactly what we have to surrender into.

Through the many names of mugwort we can learn about her medicine. Her Latin name, *Artemisia vulgaris*, is deeply connected to the Greek moon goddess Artemis. Born of Leto and the twin lunar sister of Apollo, Artemis was the sun god. After she was born, Artemis turned to aid her mother to birth her brother. The plant that was named after this bringer of relief in childbirth is still known for its use during childbirth, and with expert supervision can be used as a tea in the later stages of birth to assist with "bringing down the baby".

The dark green of the upper part of the leaves and the light silvery hue of the underside reflect the dark and light of the moon. The moon journeys with us throughout our menstrual cycles, or rather we respond to her journey as menstruating beings. This could certainly have been more relevant when there was less electric lighting and the fluctuating light of the moon would have affected hormonal cycles even more strongly. The moon provides a cyclical nature to all our lives, and offers constant companionship.

Mugwort's incredible plant spirit is reflected in the moon, the archetype of the enchantress, the capable, the protectress, the huntress, the midwife. Her namesake Artemis is often depicted riding on her horse with her bow and arrow, the epitome of strength on a knife-edge of sanity.

REASON FOR INCLUSION

Mugwort is a gateway herb, opening portals. Mugwort takes us by the hands and whispers, "Come on, come away to the land of imagination and dreams." We can work closely with dream healing using the flying ointment, so mugwort is essential in the mix in order to work with and remember our dreams, and to help develop our psychic skills.

FOLKLORE

Mugwort is said to have derived its common name from having been used to flavour drink, specifically beer drunk from a mug. So it is the wort or herb of the mug!

Like herbs such as ground ivy, it was used for brewing and flavouring beer before the introduction of hops. For this purpose, the plant was gathered when in flower and then dried. Malt liquor was then boiled with it so as to form a strong decoction, and the liquid thus prepared was added to the beer.

Another theory is that its name may come from the ancient Greek word *moughte*, meaning a moth or maggot. Along with wormwood, the plant has been regarded as useful in warding off the attacks of moths.

The Nine Herbs Charm

Known as *waremodh* ("aware-mood"), mugwort was the primary herb in the "Nine Herbs Charm", an Anglo-Saxon incantation recorded in the 10th century *Lacnunga* (Book of Remedies). Here are a few lines:

Remember, Mugwort, what you made known,

What you arranged at the Great proclamation.

You were called Una, the oldest of herbs,

you have power against three and against thirty,

you have power against poison and against infection,

you have power against the loathsome foe roving through the land.

FLY AGARIC

Latin name
Amanita muscaria

Family
Amanitaceae/amanita

Astrological ruler
Moon

Vibe
Storytelling

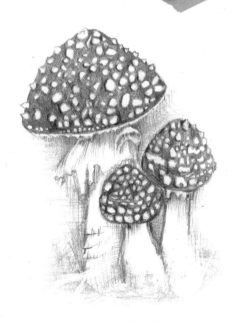

THE MAGICAL INGREDIENTS OF THE FLYING OINTMENT

MEDICINE

Images of this beautiful red and white mushroom appear in many fairy stories. Red is a powerful colour, and intrinsically attention-grabbing. Our prehistoric ancestors saw red as the colour of fire and blood, energy and primal life forces. Most of red's symbolism today arises from its powerful associations in the past. So, this mushroom attracts *everybody's* attention, and stimulates an energetic, possibly creative response – and that is just from looking at it.

Fly agaric affects us profoundly in other ways too, most notably through its interactions with our neurotransmitters. It's time for some more science ... Gamma-Aminobutyric acid (GABA) is the primary inhibitory neurotransmitter in the brain (it reduces the activity of brain neurons) and the principal neurotransmitter associated with fly agaric ingestion because fly agaric synthesizes ibotenic acid and muscimol, which structurally resembles GABA. (Both ibotenic acid and muscimol are psychoactive and can be poisonous.)

Some researchers believe that GABA controls the fear or anxiety we experience when neurons are overexcited, and GABA supplementation is therefore often used in the treatment of stress, anxiety and sleep disorders. In fact, the earliest drug ever created from the fungus in 1977 was the anxiolytic Gaboxadol. Much later in 1996, it was harnessed as a sedative.

This indicates a role for fly agaric in the reduction of fear and anxiety, which is an area we have harnessed this medicine in our practice, where we call on this polka-dotted dancer to support with:

* moving through fears
* pacifying a fear of change
* creating deeper connections with others
* exploring constructed stories within our lives
  so we can change our own narratives
* inspiring creativity for writing and creative pursuits
* sleep
* blurred vision
* chronic fatigue

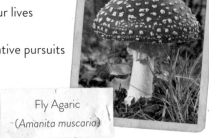

Fly Agaric
(Amanita muscaria)

REASON FOR INCLUSION

The mythical mushroom, the fly agaric, has long been associated with shamanic practices in Siberia. However, it grows commonly and prolifically in our local woodlands here in Britain and has a rich history of use in these native lands. There has been a recent resurgence in the therapeutic use of this mushroom among the herbalists of Britain, and we have also embraced this magical colourful mushroom in our work and practice.

This beautiful mushroom is a fairy-tale underground messenger offering a glimpse of some of the secrets waiting to be told. Shrouded in story and fable, this fungi brings poetic trance to the flying ointment.

FOLKLORE

The shamans, or medicine people, of Siberia make a preparation of the dried mushroom called *mukhomor*, which is imbibed to speak to their gods. They have been utilizing the *Amanita muscaria* for recreational or ritualistic purposes for centuries. At their midwinter festivals of renewal, the shaman gathers the fly agaric from under sacred trees, wearing special attire that consists of red and white fur-trimmed coats and long black boots. Pine trees, snow, flying reindeer and someone wearing red and white fur-trimmed coats – remind you of anyone?

The fly agaric has been synonymous with myth and culture for millennia, possibly one of the earliest entheogens (psychoactive substances) utilized by humans. There is so much folklore associated with this wonderful fungus that it is hard to imagine it hasn't held great importance in the development of culture and sacred worship in the past.

THE CHORUS

Last but not least, we invite our "chorus" of marshmallow, yarrow, dandelion, fennel, St John's wort and rose to bring in sweet melodies. They bring gifts of nourishment and assist in a safe and fruitful flight by providing support and care, and encouraging balance both in the flying ointment formula and its use.

MARSHMALLOW

Latin name
Althaea officinalis

Common names
Sweet weed

Plant family
Malvaceae/mallows

Astrological ruler
Venus

Vibe
Invoking healing

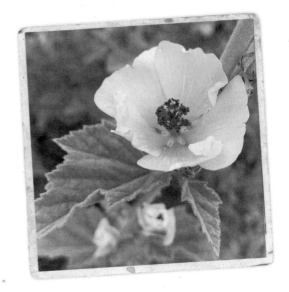

MEDICINE
The velvet-leaved, statuesque marshmallow plant is soothing and softening, and has been used for centuries to alleviate any heat in the system, including irritations of the lungs, gut, skin and mucous membranes. The plant does this through its mucilaginous qualities, which will soothe irritated or inflamed mucous membranes – a fabulous quality to have alongside herbs that can create a sense of severe dryness, as is the case with the witching herbs.

REASON FOR INCLUSION
Marshmallow can gift gentleness and nurture to all. Marshmallow medicine is all about being soft and kind to yourself; it often takes great bravery and strength of character to remember to nurture and provide for yourself as well as others.

FOLKLORE

The Greek deity Althea is a goddess of healing, marshmallow's genus' namesake. *Althaea* is from the Greek word *Althos*, meaning healing, or from *Aletheia*, meaning truth. She is a mediator who stands up for those being persecuted and believes that loving acts will bring hope into the darkest of places.

Althea saved her son from the fate dealt to him by the Fate Atropos, who decreed that once the last piece of wood in the hearth was ashes, Althea's son would die. So Althea extinguished the fire and hid the last singed piece of wood to avoid being burned to ash. Many years later, when her son murdered her brothers in a fit of rage, she brought out the piece of wood and burned it to cinders, thus extinguishing his life. Distraught, she then took her own life. In both instances, she acted in strength – first as a protector of her son and then as a protector of truth and honour.

YARROW

Latin name
Achillea millefolium

Common names
Nosebleed, old man's pepper,
soldier's woundwort, knight's
milfoil, *herbe militaris*

Plant family
Asteraceae/daisy

Astrological ruler
Mercury

Vibe
Protection

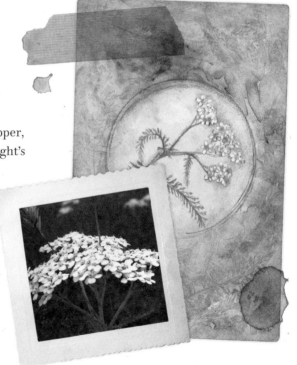

MEDICINE

Yarrow opens up blood vessels by relaxing the muscle surrounding them. It encourages circulation and movement of blood through the body.

Yarrow is high in volatile oils called azulenes, which are physically protective against pathogens. Interesting, wherever there is a physiological action of a herb for protection, such as against pathogens, this will usually point to its historical use for psychic or spiritual protection too.

REASON FOR INCLUSION

The protective and circulatory qualities of yarrow mean that wherever you are emotionally opened up when using the ointment, you can feel safe through the energy that yarrow brings. A plant of the daisy family, yarrow looks a little bit like a parasol in its morphology, which conjures up an image of its protective canopy. This strongly protective plant offers a cloak of defence, protecting the magician from psychic, energetic and physical attacks. Our mentor Christopher Hedley has described yarrow's magic for patching up open or damaged areas in the auric field.

FOLKLORE

Yarrow holds a story in its botanical name, *Achillea millefolium*. The genus name is gifted from Achilles the great warrior, hero and Greek demigod. Achilles was taught about healing arts and archery by the centaur Chiron, and he is said to have given yarrow to his soldiers to stop the bleeding from their wounds. Indeed, yarrow is a "styptic" when applied externally, meaning that it is a medicine used to staunch the flow of blood.

Achilles was a hero of the Trojan War and the greatest warrior ever seen. The legend goes that his mother, Thetis, dipped the infant Achilles into the River Styx to grant him immortality and invulnerability. She held him by his heel, not wanting to fully let go, and as a result she left Achilles' heel vulnerable. Eventually it led to his demise. He was finally killed by Paris, who shot him in his heel with an arrow. Nowadays, we all understand the term Achilles' heel to mean a point of weakness in our physicality or constitution. It can also be where we are emotionally vulnerable. Yarrow helps us to answer the key question of ourselves: where are we vulnerable and why?

The word *millefolium* means "thousand leaf", referring to the many leaflets on the finely divided leaves. The usual English name "yarrow" is apparently derived from *gearwe*, an Anglo-Saxon word meaning "well" or "enough".

DANDELION

Latin name
Taraxacum officinale

Common names
Bitterwort, blow-ball, cankerwort, clockflower, lion's tooth, piss-in-bed, pissinlit, priest's crown, puffball, swine's snout, telltime

Plant family
Asteraceae/daisy

Astrological ruler
Jupiter and the sun

Vibe
Grounding – keeping a thread to this world

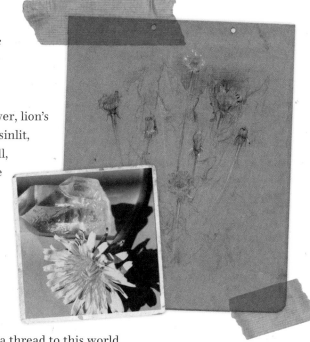

MEDICINE
The use of dandelions in the healing arts goes so far back that tracing its history is like trying to catch a dandelion seed as it floats over the grass. For millennia, people have been making tonics and teas from this herb, which can be prescribed for a huge range of ailments – from simple warts to cancer.

We use dandelion to shift and support digestion issues but also more poetically to get to the root of an issue.

REASON FOR INCLUSION

The taproot of the dandelion grows deep and strong, sometimes reaching up to 15 feet into the soil, with a tenacious spirit that helps us to keep rooted to the Earth. With the flying ointment offering us a doorway to astral projection and whizzing away to explore other realms, we include the humble dandelion in the mix to keep a thread of connection to the world we inhabit. Dandelion grows globally, helping to detoxify the planet and people who drink the liver- and kidney-cleansing plant.

Herbs grow where they are needed and this one loves to grow around spaces that need rewilding and reconnection with nature. Many people mistakenly believe that they need to irradiate dandelions from gardens and lawns, but dandelions are actually brilliant for lawns as they fertilize the grass. Their roots loosen hard-packed soil, aerating the ground and helping to reduce erosion. The deep taproot pulls up nutrients such as calcium from deep in the soil and makes them available to other plants.

We add dandelion into the mix to stabilize the ointment by bringing that deep grounded energy of the herb.

FOLKLORE

Dandelions are, quite possibly, one of the most successful plants that exist. These familiar friends are masters of survival. They can take root in places that seem short of miraculous, with tiny amounts of soil. They are super-fast growers and their blooms' life cycles from bud to seed can pass in just a few days, but the individual plants can live for many years. They can regenerate from any part of the taproot left in the ground after you have dug a harvest.

We see this plant as a perfect illustration of elemental balance. The root represents the Earth and supporting our own internal Earth in our digestive system. Dandelion leaves represent water and, being a diuretic, the plant works directly with the urinary system of our internal water, encouraging flow.

The flowers look like the sun and bring warmth with the Fire element. The seeds are the Air, connecting into our thoughts and imaginations. Legend says that blowing the seeds off a dandelion is said to carry your thoughts and dreams to your loved one.

Dandelions are named after lions, because their lion-toothed leaves can help to heal so many ailments, great and small: baldness, dandruff, toothache, sores, fevers, rotting gums, weakness, bladder infections, heart disease, lethargy and depression. So many diseases are actually caused by vitamin deficiencies and these power-packed weeds have more vitamin A than spinach, more vitamin C than oranges or tomatoes and are rich in iron, calcium and potassium.

FENNEL

Latin name
Foeniculum vulgare

Common names
Fenkel, sweet fennel, wild fennel

Plant family
Apiaceae or Umbelliferae/
carrot family

Astrological ruler
Mercury

Vibe
Balance and clear
communication

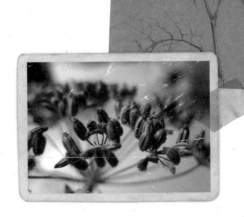

MEDICINE

Fennel is a calming digestive, balancing blood sugars and has an uplifting yet gently calming and balancing influence on the nervous system. It can be used to encourage lactation as a galactagogue and can reduce colic in an infant. And it tastes delicious too!

REASON FOR INCLUSION

Fennel holds our nerves and guts safe and sound while undertaking flight with the ointment, so it plays an essential role in helping to keep us in balance. Our intentions in the creation and utilization of the balm are also aided by the addition of this mercurial herb, which gives us space for clarity in all our communications relating to this potent medicine.

FOLKLORE

Folklore about fennel states that if you carry an amulet of this aromatic plant, people will trust you and trust your words. So it can be drawn upon in situations where you need to express words of utmost importance, such as in a job interview or a court appearance.

Fennel's most famous myth is that of the Greek Titan Prometheus, who took an ember from Olympus and hid it in the stalk of fennel, sneaking the gift of fire to humans against the wishes of the gods. His stalk of fennel held the prized contraband. So for us mortals, fire was gifted us through this lofty herb. As punishment, it was decreed that Prometheus should suffer for eternity but Zeus was unsatisfied with this and unleashed Pandora with her box of woes on humankind. Fennel brought us fire, communication and equilibrium against the odds, and the ancient curses of Zeus have been balanced by hope – the last thing left in Pandora's box.

ST JOHN'S WORT

Latin name
Hypericum perforatum

Common names
Grace of God, amber, barbe de Saint-Jean, demon chaser, goatweed

Plant family
Hypericaceae/hypericum family

Astrological ruler
Sun

Vibe
Rising upward, solar energies

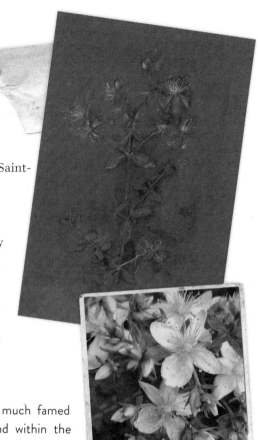

MEDICINE

This wild and abundant weed is much famed for being an anti-depressant, and within the bright yellow flowers lies a blood-red pigment signifying the alchemical action within the medicine of hypericum. It also signifies the supportive medicine of the herb, for hypericum is a wonderful wound healer (vulnerary).

The plant has the power to lift up our spirits and protect us from dark and malignant forces that may originate within our own minds and souls. For centuries, the possessed or insane inhaled the scent of the crushed leaves and flower or drank a potion made from the plant in an attempt to rid themselves of madness.

REASON FOR INCLUSION

Hypericum helps us rise up and overcome any adversity. As we are opening up to unseen forces with the magic of the flying ointment, we have included this prized medicinal herb in the mix to bolster, elevate and protect our psyches.

Hypericum is sometimes called herb of sunshine, and we want to invite its all-powerful solar energy into the potion, giving a pure and seemingly inexhaustible energy for life and light and warmth.

FOLKLORE

In global mythology, this plant is associated with the sun. In Greece, Hyperion, Helios' father, is the sun god who drove his golden chariot across the sky between dawn and dusk. In Teutonic mythology, St John's wort is dedicated to the sun god Baldur. The yellow flowers bloom around Midsummer Day. Pre-Christian Europeans celebrated midsummer at the summer solstice as an important festival of light and fire. The early Christian Church scorned all pagan worship, but they couldn't control it. When leaders of the Church discovered that St John the Baptist was born on Midsummer Day, they renamed the "Feast of Fires" as the "Feast of St John", and made 24 June St John's Day; thus the plant became known as St John's wort. The Church declared the plant sacred to St John, who had blessed it with healing power.

The doctrine of signatures, a medieval theory that God has stamped a mark on all plants to give us clues as to their uses, shows us that within the structure of the plant we can detect the sun. Light shines through the tiny translucent glands on the leaves and flowers, making them appear as miniature suns. The bright golden flowers themselves represent solar brilliance.

St John's wort has great protective powers. Gathered on Midsummer Eve, this plant can ward off dangers and mischiefs, imps, dark forces, evil spirits and the demons of melancholy.

ROSE

Rose essential oil is the very last ingredient added to the flying ointment. Garden cultivation of roses began 5,000 years ago in Asia. She truly is an ancient ancestor; fossil evidence ages her at 35 million years old. This most wonderful of plants has been a symbol of love, beauty, war and politics down the ages.

We have chosen rose for her magical ability to induce relaxation and a sense of calm love. Studies have shown that simply looking at a bunch of roses creates a relaxation response. Rose essential oil is similarly relaxing and mildly sedative. It has antiseptic and anti-inflammatory effects on the physical body, and makes a brilliant supportive tonic for the heart in times of intensity. The gently uplifting and relaxing scent of this flower reminds us of safety and security, and helps all who anoint themselves release any stresses with a sigh of relief. The rose is both gentle, loving and nourishing, and fully armed with protective barbed thorns.

Rose essential oil is highly coveted and much loved, both for its aroma and its healing benefits. The essential oil used in the flying ointment is made from extracts of the *Rosa damascena* blossom and is one of the most valued of all the oils and extremely expensive. This is because organic rose production and the process of oil extraction involve high costs. It takes 60,000 roses per ounce of oil; that works out at over 20,000 roses for just 10ml! Rose oil is the perfect scent for our flying ointment, offering heart nurture.

– 13 –
PREPARING THE
FLYING OINTMENT

The cast of performing plant players – from our three stars and their harmonies to the supportive chorus – all play their own important roles. We have studied their magical and medical qualities, and the folklore that surrounds them. It is nearly time to make the flying ointment itself using the recipe that we have perfected over the years since that serendipitous encounter with Mary in the lanes of Cornwall. First, though, we must harvest and prepare the herbs ...

HARVESTING HERBS

When harvesting any herb, conscious awareness is key, and in particular when harvesting poisonous herbs we counsel a good dose of personal responsibility. Remember that these plants have the potential to kill and thus need a little extra respect if you are cutting stems, or getting sap on your hands. It is completely your choice whether you wear gloves or not when handling the witching herbs, but note the fact that compounds from these beauties will pass through your skin and you will feel effects.

Also, any sharp blades you have used to cut your herbs should be carefully and fully cleaned before you chop your dinner vegetables with them!

Make sure your drying herbs are safely away from other people, who might make themselves teas or nibble on leaves, not knowing that these are poisonous.

The optimum times to harvest your herbs are as follows, with observations to astrological and biodynamic principles:

* Pick the herb on a dry day when the dew has disappeared from the plant.
* The aerial parts (above ground) should be harvested around the full moon.
* Harvest the roots on the new moon, when the energy is down in the Earth.

Plants' structures vary greatly, and how they are harvested is influenced by this. Harvesting the plants is part of the process of getting to know them. For example, when harvesting rosehips, they will inevitably spike you with their thorns, but usually only after you have a fair harvest, as if they are saying, "That's enough!" In comparison, elderflowers can often be picked by snapping the stem at an axis. They come clean off in a very satisfactory fashion, but need to be carefully dried and there also needs to be an effort to process them afterwards. They are giving, but then demanding of your time and effort.

HERB DRYING
You can dry herbs in a variety of ways, such as by lying them on newspaper in the airing cupboard or in a dehydrator or low temperature in the oven, or simply tied in bunches and hang up to dry.

Lavender stems will tie together nicely and create the most uplifting and calming of scents as they dry in the bedroom or living room of your home. Mugwort can be hung in fat bunches over a sheet so any flowers or leaves that fall are caught. Bunches of elderflower can be laid out on the newspaper and dried in an airing cupboard. All our washing smells of various aromatic herbs; we love it!

HERB STRIPPING
When it comes to processing your plants so that they can be stored in darkened glasses for future uses, the processing becomes its own beautiful ritual – stripping the herb from the stems.

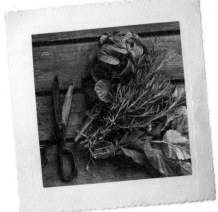

231

When commercial dried herbs are prepared, the plant material is processed through a chopping machine, which means you may get sharp stems and stalks. When you harvest and prepare a herb yourself, you can be more precise and careful with the parts of the plant you use and how you prepare them. Like us, you can take the leaves and flowers from the stalks to store and use.

Divination with Stalks

Once dried, stalks can be made into a divinatory tool. You can do this with the dried stems of yarrow and lavender in particular. When the herbs have been dried and stripped of their straight stems, gather around 40–50 of the stems and cut them to 7.5–10cm (3–4in) in length. These stems can be thrown onto a clear, stable surface and the patterns and shapes in which they fall can be read by using your intuition.

We like to hold the stripping ritual with a pipe of mugwort (see pages 78–9), and set our intentions in order to make careful observations of how each plant reacts to being worked with. You will see different feelings and responses that arise when working with different herbs in this way, all of which inform our understanding of the plant in question. We can tap into all of our senses to intuit and collect information about each plant's character and medicine.

When your fingers slide down the long lengths of lavender and work the purple aromatic buds and blooms off the top, you may discover the ends are surprisingly sharp and they do not want to give up the flowers too easily.

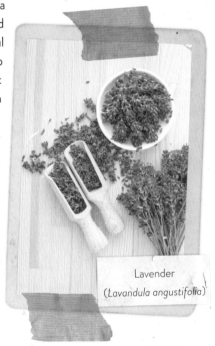

Lavender
(*Lavandula angustifolia*)

Teasing the tiny elderflowers off their individual stalks leaves your now bright-yellow hands covered in a complete dusting of silky soft pollen.

Crushing peppermint leaves as they come away from their stems infuses the air with uplifting opening scents and you notice the little bits of leaf that simply don't want to come away from the stems!

Each plant has its own individual signature and teaches us more about themselves in this practical exercise. Why not put some music on and create your own herb-processing meditation?

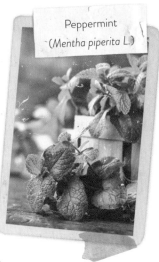

Peppermint
(Mentha piperita L.)

COMMUNITY COHESION IN RITUAL

The power plants inspire creativity and community cohesion: planting, tending, harvesting, processing, making remedies and applying these remedies can all be seen as community rituals, deepening our connection to the land, to the spirits of the herbs and to each other.

Our intentions when creating the flying ointment have always been, and always will be, to encourage a deeper connection with nature, to open up to the world with new eyes, and explore health on a personal and planetary level.

We feel called to revive and maintain this ancient native knowledge and power. Flying ointment is a tool of magic, long associated with meetings of wild wanton women wanking under the moon (and we mean wanking, rather than the censorious connotations of the term "masturbation", originally meaning "to defile"), around a fire, revelling in the pure life-force of sexual energy, the balm lovingly applied, granting astral flight and pure pleasure.

The plants give us permission to express our feral inventiveness and imagination. They support our move toward a new vision for healthcare and medicine embracing resourceful outlets and exploration, with an acceptance of the magic of nature as the norm.

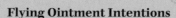

Flying Ointment Intentions

In creating the flying ointment, we visualize a social and global shift of positive change – interwoven with ceremony and creativity, both of which are held within the ointment.

We aim for grassroots "gentle" connections – re-storying a blissful healthy future, of responsibility within community.

We seek sensory herbal evolution, cultivating change through resourcefulness and play.

The commanding spirits of the plants and fungi have the gift of healing on a profoundly emotional level and also on a community level, connecting us through ritual and shared experience. They also help us to shift the collective consciousness, which has often become terrified to even hear the words "magic" or "witchcraft" uttered. As we make the preparations for each annual batch of the balm, we focus on the idea of "responsibility within community".

The ceremony of the creation of the flying ointment follows a fractal, spiralling pattern. We sit in a circle of souls, all dreaming of unity and peace. Each annual ritual is held close to the winter solstice.

Partakers are asked to prepare for it for a few days beforehand through focusing their consciousness by thinking about and writing down their reflections on the words "witch" and "ritual". A prerequisite for participants on our native power plant courses is a written piece. It always feels very poignant and powerful to witness people talking about what these words mean or represent to them. As they speak of what magic and the natural world are to them as individuals, something often seems to shift within the group. The information that comes back to us each time makes it apparent that people connect deeply to the idea, belief or philosophy of magic. Plants connect us in a practical way with the energy flowing through all of nature – the plant world and the human experience.

The preparation for each annual ceremony follows the herbs through the 13 moons of the year, planting and harvesting them at optimum times. Each new batch of the base oil includes a few drops of oil from the previous one. This has been a recurring pattern for many years, carrying the hopes and intentions of hundreds of people into each batch of balm. When we create a green oil base for our medicinal flying ointment during these sessions, there is always a sense of community coming together to celebrate and tap into ancient practices.

The creation of the remedy includes making an infused oil preparation. Some of the plant material is added to this throughout the cycle of the year when it is ready to harvest, so some of the dried plant materials are macerated in the almond oil for as long as 13 moons. During this time the glass jar filled with this oil is left out in the sunshine and full moon rays to gain blessing from these celestial bodies.

Other herbs are gathered over the year, and dried in preparation for the next circular rite. On the final day, herbs are added by each individual to the already green oil and made into a hot oil preparation. Warming the oil draws out the ingredients' fat-soluble chemical constituents. Words of community cohesion and responsibility are also added to the oils with each plant and stirred into the pot.

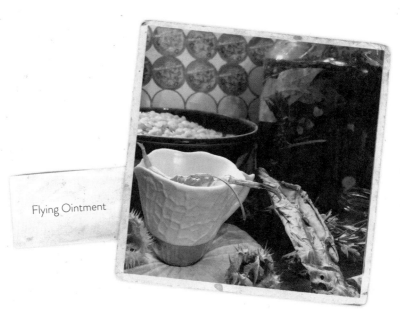

Flying Ointment

RECIPE FOR THE FLYING OINTMENT

To make a flying ointment the first thing you must possess is patience. This is not a preparation for which you can buy all the ingredients on the internet or from a local shop. This is about dedication to nature and to Spirit, and that takes attention to detail and the most precious commodity – time.

Each of the plants in this recipe can be grown or sought out in the wild and befriended; and when you do this your potion shall have potency and you shall have the power to wield and create strong magic.

The conversation and relationship with the land is paramount. Create your soil, feed the compost heap, encourage the worm population in your garden and invite fertility and diversity into and onto the land. Ask the heavens and the stars for seeds, hold the idea of what you want to create in your mind's eye and talk to the cosmic forces about your vision. Sometimes the plants will simply turn up if you welcome them with an open heart and enquiring soul.

The creation of the flying ointment is a cyclical spell – from planting the seeds to harvesting at the most auspicious moments.

Steps:

1. On the darkest moon in January, collect a 15cm (6in) length of thick mandrake root.
2. Place the root on a wooden chopping board and chop it finely. As you do, sing to it, thanking the plant for this sacrifice.
3. Place the chopped roots into a heat-proof glass bowl and cover with three cups of oil.
4. Add a teaspoon of soot to the oil.

5. Sit the glass in a cauldron half full of spring water so that the glass sits above the water like a bain-marie. Heat the water to a gentle simmer and keep it low for nine hours, so that the oil never heats so much that the root becomes cooked. All moisture must have evaporated out of the oil to ensure it will keep well.

6. On the Taurean moon in February, sing to your glass jar of mandrake-and-soot oil, asking for positive energy and only good vibes in your potion.

7. On the new moon at the Equinox in March or early April, dig up a large, fat dandelion root. Chop your root and whisper words of tenacity. Thank Jupiter and dandelion for their guidance and elemental dynamisms.

8. Leave your chopped dandelion root out in the early spring sunlight for five hours. Bring the dandelion root inside and warm next to the fire. When your dandelion root is bone dry, add the pieces into the mandrake-and-soot oil on a Virgo moon, holding thoughts of staying rooted while creating and using your oil.

9. When the moon transits Capricorn take your oil out and reflect on your own community and what you bring to it. The dandelion brings a quality of Capricorn and staying true to your word.

10. On the Beltane full moon in May, sit in the moonlight, hold the glass jar in your lap and speak your needs into the jar.

11. On the full moon at the summer solstice, at around midday, carefully pick 30 yellow flowers of hypericum. Place the oil on a table under the moon and in full solar heat for three days and nights, adding the hypericum flowers to this daily, with a song to the sun for power.

12. When the moon next transits through Leo, bring out the oil and sing or play your most lively music to bring a sense of fire and passion to the oil.

13. On the July full moon, harvest 13 datura flowers, 13 henbane leaves and 13 flowers, 2cm (1in) of aconite root, 13 belladonna

leaves and 13 flowers and 13 marshmallow leaves. Place them all back into the glass bowl with all your magical oil poured over the top. Set the bowl or bain-marie over simmering spring water in the cauldron, and re-infuse the oil with all of these lunar cycle herbs using the heat method. It will take another nine hours until all the herbs are dry but not smoky and burned. As the brew simmers and creates, whisper words of connection and revelations to the pot from time to time. Add a little extra oil if needed to cover the herbs at any point during the creation of the green oil.

14. Over the next lunar cycle, observe when the moon enters the astrological signs listed below and add to the oil to draw in energy linked to the corresponding herb with each sign. Each herb added to the mix brings qualities that will offer power to the magic, enhanced by the lunar energy:

* Scorpio moon: datura for embracing your sexuality and the ability to shape shift
* Sagittarius moon: henbane for celebration of death and endings and the new beginnings created in their wake
* Aquarius moon: aconite for flight, astral projection and for adding inspiration for thoughts and ideas to the preparation
* Aries moon: belladonna for cutting ties to unhelpful connections and to bring the determination to do this
* Cancerian moon: marshmallow leaf for invoking healing and care to support and stabilize your magical work

15. On the August full moon, harvest a small bunch of mugwort flowers and three flowering tops of yarrow. Lay these on paper for three days in a warm place to dry before adding to the oil. Cover with a lid.
16. On the next Pisces moon ask for the mugwort to support your dreaming practices.

17. On the next Gemini moon, bring out your oil again and focus on the yarrow, which will gift protection in all magical practices carried out using the flying ointment.

18. On the Equinox September full moon, the time for seed harvest is upon us. Harvest three heads of fennel seeds and dry for five days or until the next Gemini moon. Add the seeds to your oil to bring clear and necessary communications, along with wishes that your magic will permeate out and reach all those in need of it. The fennel brings balance and inspiration for how to best use this potion for nurture, love and to benefit all of life in our Universe.

19. At the end of September/early October, on the lunar equinox, there will be a Scorpio moon either on or just after the dark moon. This is the potent time to harvest the seed head of the night beauty – datura. This unraveller of the internal world and shapeshifting power plant will add an air of mystery and personal exploration into the mix; she will bring a sense of freedom and unleashed sexual energy. The seed pod can be fully dried and opened to let all the dark seeds burst out. Add these to the oil.

20. Just over a week after the Scorpio moon, the waxing moon will be in Pisces. Fly agaric adorns the woodlands – ready to tell your story, to change the story and to bring gifts from the underworld and storyland. Harvest three of these toadstools, preferably with still closed caps, and slice to dry them swiftly in a warm dry place. This will avoid maggot infestation. As you add the dried slices to the oil, think of the stories you tell and how this can carry your magic out into the hearts and minds of others.

21. Just before the November dark moon, when the moon transits Libra, go and find rose thorns. Pick five thorns, add to the oil and place on the lid. These provide grandmotherly matriarchal protection. To know when enough is enough.

22. During the December lunar cycle revisit the jar regularly, recognizing and appreciating the power

and magic of its contents. Sing or hum over it and
be grateful for the plethora of gifts that await.

23. At the January full moon, it is time to strain your oil and prepare
to make the balm. The green oil can be stored but we suggest
making a pot at a time to work with. The following recipe is for
a 60g (2oz) jar which is a large quantity of this potent mix.
You may want to make four pots with 15g (0.5oz) jars. This
is a powerful prescription for magic, connection, nature and
acceptance, and does not need to be made readily available in vast
quantities. And the balm can go rancid if left unused over time.

For the balm you will need:

* 32ml (1.5 tbsp) green oil
* 16g (1 tbsp) cocoa butter
* 8g (½ tbsp) beeswax
* 10 drops of rose essential oil

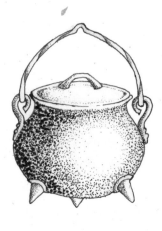

Steps:

1. Melt the cocoa butter and
beeswax into the green oil over
your cauldron bain-marie.
2. When it looks melted together, wait another ten
minutes longer to ensure it has all fully melted.
3. Take from the heat, add the essential oil and pour
immediately into a 60g (2oz) jar or four 15g (0.5oz) jars.

- 14 -
GETTING READY TO FLY

hysical and energetic protection are important considerations when using the flying ointment. When altering your state of consciousness – whether through alcohol, nicotine or any range of psychotropics – you can support your journey by considering:

* which herbs or substances might support you, such as taking milk thistle for liver protection or valerian for nerve protection.
* whether to eat or fast beforehand, and how this is likely to affect you physically and mentally. (Be aware that fasting always creates more intense experiences.)
* what additions may make the experience more memorable or smooth. For example, if you are inside do you want to burn certain oils or incenses?
* what is the ideal atmosphere, including the location, light sources, surrounding colours and safety procedures? Are you in nature, and is there enough time before sundown to get yourself ready?
* your state of mind: what are your intentions going into the experience?

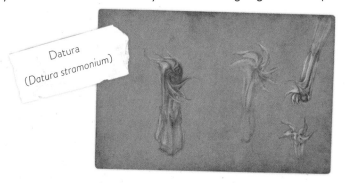

Datura
(Datura stramonium)

When getting ready to fly with the ointment, create your own flight plan that addresses magical factors as well as mundane practicalities.

* Ensure an atmosphere of loving-care is created.
* Work from a position of consideration, with clear intention. Cast a circle of energetic protection. Using a visualization of a protective orb or something physical like salt around you. See casting a circle on page 44.
* Give a nod to the moon in reverence.
* Invite in the elements: water for cleansing and hope, fire for passion and love, air for inspiration and clear communication, and earth for staying connected to the Earth.

As your flying ointment should ideally be created in support of ritual, connection and play, there will already be a sense of intention before it is utilized. It focuses the mind and places conscious awareness around the whole preparation of the ointment and its use.

READYING THE BODY FOR TAKE-OFF

Let us protect the physical body through combining herbs that synergize and support each other. Let us protect the nerves as well as the mucous membranes, kidneys and liver.

MILK THISTLE, *CARDUUS MARIANUM*

This robust, spiky, beautiful thistle holds and protects our work with the flying ointment. By supporting the liver, an organ of elimination and cleansing, the milk thistle offers fortification in any magical work with the flying ointment. Milk thistle assists the excretion of excess toxins by the liver. The super-spiky seed heads grant a suit of armour so that we are free to work in non-ordinary realities knowing that milk thistle has us protected physically and energetically.

This milky-leaved thistle was once famed for supporting breastfeeding mothers. The doctrine of signatures indicates that the milky white veins that run through the plant's leaves offer support with milk production. This herb is an excellent galactagogue (milk promoter), which gave rise to its common name.

We have been growing and harvesting the spiky seed pods for many years as we love the beneficial effects. The nutty, nutritious, dark brown seeds can help the liver regenerate four times faster than normal.

Milk thistle has also been shown to lower blood lipids, helping with emotional stability and increasing the flow of bile from the liver and gall bladder. It helps to prevent and reverse liver damage, and reduces the fatty degeneration of the liver. The herb acts on the membranes of liver cells, preventing the entry of toxic substances; thus damage to liver cells is prevented. The plant in full purple flower is extremely regal in appearance and gives the impression of an impenetrable fortress.

Fastening the seatbelt ready for take-off can be achieved through ingestion of milk thistle seeds to aid with detoxification, and to bring an element of safeguarding, both strengthening and shielding magical work.

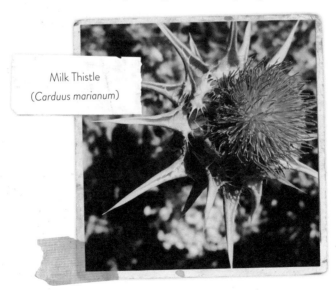

Milk Thistle
(*Carduus marianum*)

INVOCATION TO MILK THISTLE

When taking milk thistle as part of your preparations for flying with the ointment, invoke the spirit of the plant for added protection:

With a focus on health,

we invite

the highly armoured

and most protective regal plant

milk thistle

to bring protection

to this highly charged work.

Perfect symmetry,

Clearly defined outlined

Milk veins

Crawling toward lethal spears,

Shooting upward to meet the sun,

Regal heads crowned in glory

Danger ...

If you come questioning who you are

Protect your soft centre

Careful planning to attain the prize.

Tick-tock –

Catch me before my

Enriched rejuvenating

Medicine takes flight ...

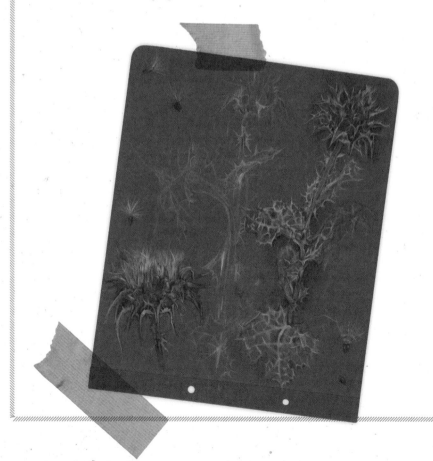

- 15 -
USING THE FLYING OINTMENT

 ow let us introduce you to a few of our favourite practices that are greatly enhanced by the use of flying ointment:

Meditation
invites us to slow down and open a channel to the subconscious mind.

Divination
asks us to pause and connect with something greater than ourselves.

Trance states
an ecstatic sweeping away of cobwebs and a heating up of energies.

Dream work
a practice that takes us deep into the unconscious.

The herbs of the flying ointment greatly support these consciousness-shifting practices, and can bring some mythologies of their own into the mix.

In preparation for all the following practices make sure that you have plenty of time: you do not want to rush around afterwards nor have to drive or operate any machinery for at least four to five hours after applying the balm.

Protecting yourself with milk thistle is always advisable, as is setting the scene by refreshing your altar space, lighting a candle and creating an intention for your work, maybe choosing some music or delighting your sense of smell with incense or essential oils.

MEDITATION

Many of us today draw on the practice of meditation for staying sane in an ever-fluctuating world. Meditation keeps us closer to balance and good health. It can support us greatly in keeping calm through various stages of chaos in our lives.

Meditation is a discipline, with countless different schools and methods. It has become popularized as enhancing relaxation, a state of focus and awareness ideally creating a sense of peace and harmony. As well as offering relaxation, meditation is a wonderful tool for encouraging and developing concentration, clarity and emotional resilience.

The Latin word for "ponder", *meditari*, is the root of the word meditate. The oldest recorded evidence of the practice of meditation is in wall art in the Indian subcontinent, dating from approximately 5,000–3,500 BCE. These images show people in the classic meditative posture with half-closed eyes that is often conjured up in the imagination whenever someone mentions the practice of meditation.

INVITE A SENSE OF FLOW TO YOUR MEDITATION

Stilling the mind is an important skill for gardeners of witching herbs and magical practitioners to cultivate, as it allows space in which to listen to our intuition more clearly, and to connect in with the power plants.

Meditation is great to practice with plants, especially the witching herbs. When the flying ointment is applied before working in the garden or plot, it can aid with calming the mundane chitter-chatter of the mind and bring a sense of clarity, connection and creativity to the fore.

Similarly, bringing a pen and paper into your garden to draw your special plants is a great way to experience deeper plant connections with them. Keen observation is often key when you draw or paint, and it is a wonderful way to let your worries drift away and to learn more about your plant friends. Applying your balm for this will add an extra special element and open up your senses to the whole experience in a more profound way.

MEDITATING WITH THE FLYING OINTMENT

Application of the flying ointment can be used alongside your existing meditative practices. Following the guidelines above by taking milk thistle and setting your intention are recommended before you begin.

Steps:

1. Apply the balm to the inner elbows.
2. Deepen your breath. Feel the energy of life-breath and life force as it moves through your physical body.
3. Understand this air is the same mixture of molecules that your ancestors inhaled and exhaled ... The same oxygen and carbon dioxide ... It has been continuously recycled since the dinosaurs walked and breathed on this Earth.
4. Allow any sensations to settle. When you are ready, finish your practice. Take note of how you feel. Leave space to relax and enjoy the sensations. Make sure you experience a reintegration with the physical world before you go about your day.

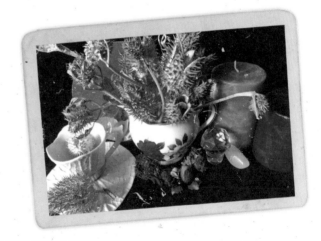

DIVINATION

The word divination originates from the Latin *divinare*, which means to foresee or foretell. It is the practice of determining the hidden significance or cause of events, and of gaining insights into the future. It is a means to connect and communicate with the divine.

Magical healers have always tapped into natural magic to find resources and seek congruence with the universal life force in their work. These divinatory practices can aid us in making important decisions. They have been sought after for centuries by people of power, many of whom employed the services of seers as aids.

The practice of the seer works on the principle that everything is interconnected on an energetic level, a web with each silken strand woven into the next. This enables access to the infinite web, where we can ask and receive answers on an unlimited basis. The herbs in the flying ointment have been used to facilitate access to the web by sorcerers, seers, psychics and witches throughout time. Psychic practices include both reading natural signs and other tools:

* cloud shapes
* patterns in the sea
* the stars
* herbal stems (and *I Ching*)
* palmistry

* astrology
* tarot
* runes
* scrying and mirror magic

When used to assist divination, the flying ointment can connect you into the timeless space, the space of the seer. Signs or visions will appear and inspirations occur. Visions may become seamlessly interpreted, certainties arise in this space and questions are answered.

This space allows for channelling of the divine, the archetypes and deities connected with the mythical history of the plants. The ointment focuses attention, enhancing the power and meaning of a divinatory reading.

249

USING THE FLYING OINTMENT FOR DIVINATION

Application of the flying ointment for the purposes of divination can be turned into a ritual of its own:

Steps:

1. Chose your method of divination and prepare yourself.
2. Write down your queries – what are you asking divine sight to reveal to you?
3. Light a candle and burn some incense to open your rite.
4. Place a small amount of your flying ointment on the pulse points of your inner wrists.
5. Call to each of the ointment plants in turn and ask for their wisdom and guidance.
6. Rub a small amount of the flying ointment onto your temples. Applying the ointment will increase awareness and perception, gift insight and promote visual acuity.
7. Start your reading.

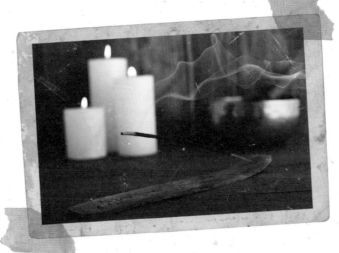

TRANCE STATES

There are lots of ways to induce trance states, ranging from self-hypnosis techniques to breath-work, but our favourite by far is that of finding ecstasy through dancing to some funky beats.

A trance dance state is a marvellous experience; a feeling of moving between the worlds of the conscious and subconscious mind. We can say farewell to the conscious mind, leaving space for the thrilling and feral part of our imagination.

Ecstatic dance has been practised throughout history and described in classical tales of Maenads dancing with the wine-god Dionysus. In the widespread practices of shamanism, ecstatic dance and rhythmic drumming are used to alter consciousness in spiritual practices. But it is in the toe-tapping footsteps of those delirious Maenads that we dance today, drawing on the energy of rave, sexy salsa, frenzied foxtrot, whirly waltz and finding our own sense of wild abandonment in boogie.

The flying ointment can connect us with fierce, unabashed ancestors when we simply stick some tunes on, vacate our minds and release ourselves to the rhythm, moving freely as the music takes us. The melody and power plants course through our blood, leading to a trance state and a feeling of ecstasy.

USING THE FLYING OINTMENT TO TRANCE DANCE

Trance dance can be an essential part of your magical practice and your mental health care regime, when you give yourself up to the tango of each and every full moon.

Steps:

1. Apply the balm to the backs of the knees and behind the ears.
2. Dance!
3. As you warm up from dancing, the balm will absorb more readily into the creases of your skin.

DREAM WORK

There are countless ideas about exactly why we dream. Many conjecture that dreaming contributes to our emotional, physical and spiritual health. We may not remember dreaming, but everyone is thought to dream between three to six times per night, with each dream lasting between five to twenty minutes. And as odd as our dreams may appear, science has shown that dreams are powerful resources for emotional resolution, and that they help us prepare for life's stresses. The pineal gland has been likened to the seat of consciousness. It becomes active when we are in deep rapid eye movement (REM) sleep, creating our dream world. The release of melatonin at night balances out the sleep–wake cycle, keeping us balanced and connected with the cycles of day and night.

One of our most mysterious and intriguing states of consciousness is in the dream state, when we dive into the deep waters of sleep. Dreams provide insights into our aspirations, hopes and fears. They can respond to our innermost wishes and desires, be a catalyst to creativity and provide us with answers to questions that have evaded us in daily life. When we dream we are not confined by the physical body, nor by time or space, so we enter into an arena beyond that of the rational mind; we enter the dream space.

The dream space is a mystical realm where, with practice, we can become lucid, aware of our dreams and even affect their outcomes. This place is one of the thin spaces, where the veils are gossamer fine and the facilitation of free movement of consciousness, magic and healing are possible.

In many cultures around the world, dreams have long had an association with healing; the ancient Greeks and Egyptians both had dream temples where people went to seek healing. Dreams are also significant to Native American cultures; they open up worlds and realms beyond our day-to-day understanding of reality. According to their traditions, "dreamwalkers" are those who work within these spaces to practise many differing kinds of medicine.

Our wise time-travelling wizard mentor, Christopher Hedley, taught us much about dream work and dream healing. When he travelled from England across the Atlantic, he was introduced to the idea that if you're working with someone or something overly challenging, you should dream on it. He also introduced us to the concept of dream amulets, which can be filled with a healing herb to assist those seeking nocturnal visions and wishing to set out on dream journeys. Herbal amulets are also known as medicine bags, power bags, mojo bags and sachet bags in different cultures. In particular, a mugwort herb amulet is a wonderful additional tool to encourage and work with your dreams.

African Traditional Dream Healing

South Africa Zulu and Xhosa traditional practices draw on the dream space to support a healing journey. The Zulu healer (*isangoma*) develops what is known as "a soft head" and becomes "a house of dreams", and is then guided to harvest and apply cleansing medicinal roots. After being directed in the liminal space to where a special healing plant can be found, the healer's next waking hours will be spent harvesting and preparing this plant for use in the treatment of their patient.

Dreams are intelligent. They can be a valuable key to uncovering unconscious process and unlocking intuition. Analysing and recording dreams can therefore offer an opportunity for the dreamer to recognize the mind's own power to heal itself. All you really need is a journal and pen to record them.

Dreams can be seen as metaphorical representations of what's going on in your subconscious. You can learn things about yourself, your past and your emotional health from your dreams. Issues that are sometimes repressed in waking life, but are seeking attention can be harnessed as healing tools.

The flying ointment can be used in dream work as a healing tool. The flying ointment includes the famous "dream herb", mugwort. However, all the psychotropic herbs contained within the mix can help to guide, enhance and aid in dream work. The power plant herbs have been documented through the ages as reliable dream-enhancing plants. The ointment can also encourage a waking dream state when used, creating more vivid and connected visions.

HOW TO MAKE A DREAM AMULET

An amulet is a type of charm, a form of sympathetic magic, that attracts positive enhancement, bringing luck and clarity in communication. They can be made with any herb and for many different types of magical connection. Here we will be focusing on mugwort to enhance your dreaming work further.

You will need:

* a piece of natural material such as cotton or silk measuring 10cm by 10cm (4in by 4in)
* a generous pinch of dried mugwort
* symbolic items such as special stones, crystals, acorn, shell, feather
* a pinch of the flying ointment balm
* a written wish (optional)
* ribbon

Steps:

1. Spread your open piece of material on your altar.
2. Place a healthy pinch of mugwort in the centre of your material.
3. Now anoint your power object(s) with a little of the flying ointment balm. As you anoint them, concentrate on your intention for your dreaming.
4. Place them on the sprinkled herb and draw up the edges of your material. Tie it up with ribbon of your colour choice.
5. Place your dream amulet by your bedside or pillow before you go to sleep at night – and dream ...
6. Record your dreams when you wake.

DREAM WORK WITH THE FLYING OINTMENT

Before you begin working with the flying ointment in dream work, it is essential that you practice dream recall. Keep a notebook by the side of your bed (or some other way of recording a dream when it occurs). Make a note of your dreams straight away as they often disappear very quickly. Keeping a consistent diary will help you to recognize recurring patterns and symbols in your dreams.

Once you have done this for at least one lunar cycle (28 days) you will be more adept at recalling your dreams regularly. Becoming connected to your dreams can alter your sense of ordinary reality; sometimes you may not even distinguish between what was dreamed and what was experienced in physical form.

To start your dreaming practice with the flying ointment follow the below steps:

1. Listen to a relaxing piece of music that you love and apply a little of the balm to your temples.
2. Set a clear intention to remember your dreams and receive insight. Perhaps there is a specific problem or issue you want clarity with.
3. Repeat the following incantation as you go to sleep: "I am open to receiving insights from my dreams."
4. When you wake, stay lying in the same position for a little while and try not to move until the dream is clear in your mind.
5. Take some time to think about the theme of your dream, how you felt and what symbols were shown before writing it down or recording it.

It can be very helpful to join a small group of people who are interested in making sense of their dreams so that you can share your dreams and help each other to understand them better.

– 16 –

SACRED SEXUALITY WITH THE FLYING OINTMENT AND PASSION POTION

"Drink all your passion and be a disgrace", from Sufi poet Rumi's poem "A Community of the Spirit", has been adopted as our mantra over the years. It reminds us to remember to engage in life and all its richness, our passion, while feeling wild and free. One of our potions in particular embodies this great line: the Passion Potion – drops of desire.

The Passion Potion Experience

There they were at dawn on a midsummer morning in the centre of an ancient yew maze, chanting these intoxicating words over and over: "drink all your passion and be a disgrace, drink all your passion and be a disgrace". Long white gowns; young, wild witchy energy. As the sun rose, they dripped searing hot chilli Passion Potion onto one another's tongues and rubbed the magical flying ointment onto their pulse points. The bright light of the sun invaded all corners of the dark maze with its morning vigour, clearing the night's fears from each nook and cranny. Only the night before when the maze had been illuminated by the cool blue tones of the moon, the horrors had been rampant. Whispy white tortured-looking figures rushed passed them and others could be seen cowering in the curves of the maze hedge. They somehow stumbled about and found their way out of the maze, and across the castle lawn back to their beds in their travelling wagons. They lay shaking, sleepless, half laughing, a nervous and thankful laugh, with moonlight providing some relief.

In the morning light, back at the centre of the maze, they'd come to face their fears. A residue remained of the feeling initiated by visions of the translucent, crouched figures from last night.

The drops of desire from the Passion Potion dripped down their chins and the chant rose in intensity as the dragon energy rose in them. Blood-hot from the chilli; the childlike daisy syrup had brought fun and joy to the overexcited mayhem, while the deep dark, dank valerian root stilled and jittery anxiety from their ghostly experience. They began to feel that they had been offered a great gift, to return to the place of fear and release the energy that had created the visions. Tripping over their gowns they ran, ran about the maze, laughing and shrieking and chanting – until they felt completely free. Free to climb higher and higher up the ancient yew that overlooked the maze. Their white gowns became filthy and their hair fell about their shoulders.

Desire totally engulfed the witches, consumed them, the love in their hearts for this ancient tree and passion for all magical nature work reached boiling point. The triplicate potion had aided their full flight to freedom, while Rumi's words have unleashed the racing beat of the Earth's song and they were helpless in the dance carried by the current of a combined dream.

The three herbs of the Passion Potion work synergistically. The fire chilli in the potion speaks of dragons lying dormant, waiting patiently for the calling. The valerian represents unleashed inhibitions and the daisy signifies childlike play all through life. Together, they stand for unbridled passions and trusting in the spirits of the elements to guide the voyage. A profound connection once felt is never forgotten, and guaranteed to be imprinted on the heart for ever.

SACRED SEXUALITY

A transcendental experience can be created through harnessing sexual desire, directing lust, experiencing self-pleasure, erotic exploration and sexual connection with others. Through eroticism and creativity with an intention to transcend the bodily encounter, we can go beyond the physical sexual experience and move into a state of delight, bliss and thrilling wonderment; an altered state.

Our Hallucino-Lube, aka the flying ointment, is infused with powerful sex magic intentions. The lube has earned a multitude of raunchy titles, including cock and cunts trippy lube, or lusty lube, among others.

The use of plants in sex rites isn't a new thing. People have been experimenting with ways to turn themselves on since the dawn of time, and notorious bath-house romps and outrageous Roman orgies are known to have had our nightshade celebrities present as part of the proceedings.

Over time, the expansive and elusive history of sex magic was further suppressed by the Christian dread of anything suggestive; thus it's often difficult to obtain records about it. In his 1970s book *Sex and the Supernatural*, Benjamin Walker writes that Urgyan, in central Asia, is perhaps where the earliest accounts of erotic sex magic can be found. Urgyan is described as a semi-mythical kingdom that fought for the rights of the Tibetan people, and where intercourse was regarded as not only for the purpose of procreation, but also for the acquisition of magical power.

INTRODUCING THE PASSION POTION

Sex can be a most charming and rousing magic, and the intimacy of revealing your intention is super-charged. Passion is fire energy, bringing creativity, electrifying fun, stimulating play and lusty desires. This is why our Passion Potion is wondrous to use in combination with the flying ointment for these spicy, sensual and heart-felt practices.

Passion Potion is also useful for any situation in which there is a lack of passion, which may potentially manifest as a lack of motivation, or no zest for life anymore. Just a few drops of the herb combination taken daily can really

CHILLI MEDICINE

What is it about chilli that makes it so exciting and addictive? The chilli rush.

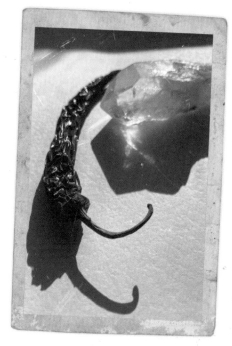

The alkaloid phytochemicals that give chilli peppers their intensity, when ingested or applied topically, are known as the capsaicinoids. Capsaicin is one of these. They are thought to be produced as secondary metabolites by the chilli peppers as deterrents against certain mammals and fungi.

When the chilli peppers are consumed by mammals, such as humans, capsaicin binds with pain receptors in the mouth and throat, evoking pain via spinal relays to the brain, where heat and discomfort are perceived. In response to the heat, our bodies produce endorphins, the feel-good hormone factors that provide pain relief. And on top of that we become flushed: our lips can become plump and luscious and before you know it you feel as if you are having a steamy moment. Senses are heightened and circulation is pumping. This intensity and sense of the "heat" of chilli peppers is officially measured in Scoville heat units.

MEDICINAL MAGIC OF CHILLI

The capsaicin in chilli has metabolism-boosting properties, helping to increase the amount of heat your body produces, thus burning more calories. It does this through a process called diet-induced thermogenesis, which causes an increase in your metabolism. Chilli is high in vitamin C, improves circulation and relieves pain. These, alongside the myriad of other health-giving properties, make chilli a great health-giving food and medicine. Chilli is even anti-viral against a host of viruses, including the shingles herpes virus.

VALERIAN THE SENSUAL

Valeriana officinalis belongs to the Caprifoliaceae, or honeysuckle, plant family. This plant has got such a powerful distinctive scent that, when freshly dug up, the aroma itself can completely alter conscious perceptions. There have been a few times when, studying valerian with groups of students, we have all lost ourselves in a sensuous space. For a few moments, we've all been high on the whiff of those spaghetti-like roots! There is no mistaking that this is strong medicine.

At the time of first making the Passion Potion, we had no idea that valerian has been traditionally used as an aphrodisiac. As we've explained, it soon became clear to us that our concoction created a powerfully erotic effect! We were curious as to why. So we went to the books to research further, thus discovering this traditional use of the spicy, smelly valerian root.

In the mix, the valerian works magic and medicine by relaxing the muscles of the body, releasing tension and therefore releasing inhibitions. The plant removes nervous tension, washing tightness, pressures and strains away. Valerian relaxes the smooth muscle of the blood vessel walls, allowing the chilli to be delivered throughout the body, thereby heightening senses at the extremities, letting the toes and fingertips feel more too.

Many people use valerian to induce sleep, which means that after an evening on the potion you shouldn't find it hard to rest. However, it doesn't generally seem to induce tiredness when taken as part of the stimulating aphrodisiac concoction that is the Passion Potion.

DAISY THE DELIGHTFUL

Daisy, or the "day's eye" (the origin of the name), is one of the first connections to the plant world that many children have. Part of the Compositae, or daisy, family of plants (all named after her), she imparts her medicine to us in our youth through her sense of play and enchantment. Who can remember making a daisy chain or plucking petals chanting "loves me, loves me not"? In the potion, the daisy brings a sense of playfulness,

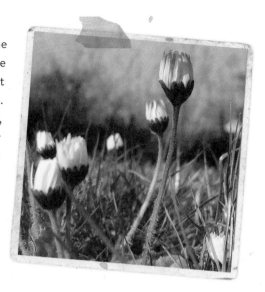

fun and joy. Guarding us from bruising – both physical and emotional – the daisy gifts a resilience and sense of possibilities, all in innocence and fun. To be free to flow in sex and the erotic, a sense of play is paramount.

MAKE YOUR OWN PASSION POTION

The passion potion has three main ingredients: chilli tincture, valerian tincture and daisy syrup, all of which can be easily made at home. As we've mentioned, magical intention really starts with growing and harvesting plants, which is why we grow our chillies lovingly in our greenhouse or on our windowsills indoors and grow valerian in our gardens (but it can be grown in pots). The daisy we wildcraft from the abundance of flowers in the summer.

We would encourage you to do the same – growing and harvesting your plants with an awareness of your magical intentions. Then, when the time is right, combine them to create your own passion potion, and enjoy ...

Here are instructions for each of the main stages.

CHILLI TINCTURE INTENTION

The first thing you will need for your Passion Potion is a chilli tincture, a hot, spicy concoction to invite some spice into your life.

Steps:

1. *Chop up around 30 fresh chillies (or enough to fill your jar), taking great care not to touch your face, eyes or genitals!*
2. *Fill a clean jam jar with the chopped chillies. Completely cover the chillies with brandy, label "Chilli Brandy for Passion Potion" and leave for a lunar cycle (28 days).*
3. *Strain the mixture by decanting it through muslin. Put aside the chillies and pour the resulting tincture into a clean jar.*
4. *Place one drop on your tongue to taste just how hot the brandy has become.*
5. *Label the jar with the name of the herb, the date, where you gathered or obtained the chillies, and what the moon was doing at the time. Chilli falls under the domain of the sun or Mars, so Leo, Aries or Scorpio moon transits will be extra powerful for working with this plant.*

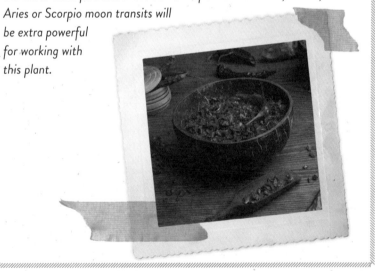

VALERIAN TINCTURE INTENTION

The next thing you will need for your Passion Potion is a valerian tincture, an earthy blend to help you release your inhibitions and agitations.

Steps:

1. Dig up the pungent roots of a mature, three-year-old valerian plant. Give the roots a rinse and chop them as small as you can.
2. Fill a jam jar with them before completely covering them with brandy – all the roots need to be properly submerged.
3. Label the jar with the words "Valerian Tincture for Passion Potion" and leave for one lunar cycle (28 days).
4. Strain the mixture through muslin, discard the root material and pour the resulting tincture back into a clean jar.
5. Label with the name of the herb, the date, where you harvested it and what the moon was doing at the time. Valerian is under the domain of Mercury, so Gemini or Virgo moon transits will have super potency for working with this plant.

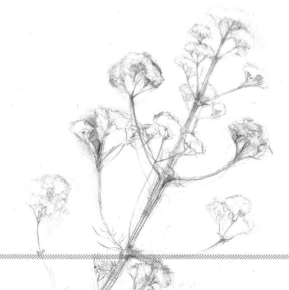

DAISY SYRUP INTENTION

The final thing you will need for your Passion Potion is a daisy syrup intention, a sweet mixture that invites playfulness and a sense of joy into your life.

Steps:

1. Harvest a small bowlful of daisy heads. Daisies fall under the domain of the sun, so Leo moon transits will have extra potency for working with this plant.
2. Place the flowers in a pan and pour water over them until they're covered.
3. Bring the daisy tea nearly to the boil and just keep under boiling temperature for a while until the water turns a lovely pale green-brown colour.
4. Sieve the daisies out when pouring the liquid into a measuring jug. Return the liquid to the pan.
5. Now add approx. 500g (1lb) of sugar per pint of the liquid in the pan and gently warm until all the sugar has dissolved.
6. Keep over the heat for a further five minutes to make sure the sugar and tea are fully incorporated.
7. Pour into sterilized bottles and label as "Daisy Syrup for Passion Potion", listing the name, date, and when and where the flowers were harvested.

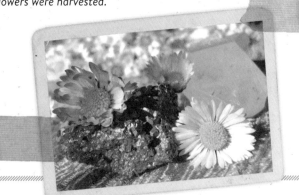

PASSION POTION RECIPE

To make a 100ml (3fl oz) bottle you will need:

* 60ml (4 tbsp) daisy syrup
* 40ml (3 tbsp) valerian tincture
* 0.5ml (approx. 10 drops) chilli tincture

Steps:

1. *Mix the daisy syrup and valerian tincture together in a small bowl.*
2. *Add the chilli tincture gradually. The strength of chilli tincture drops can be variable and also change with time, so you really need to feel your own way through the amounts. You want the chilli to come through very strongly, though, so that it can really get to work. One difficulty you may face is that after you've tasted the chilli once, you have no idea of the strength of future tastes as your tongue is already chilli-infused. You may need lots of helpers and their fresh tongues to try it out on. You know you've got enough when you can really feel it and react with something like, "Wow, that's got a kick!"*

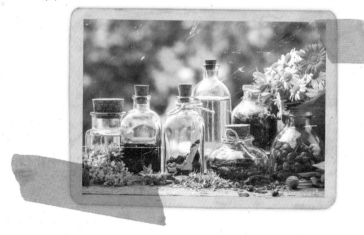

SACRED RITES WITH THE BALM AND PASSION POTION

Sex and pleasure are utterly sacred states, and harnessing the power of orgasm for healing is very much part of the power of the witch archetype – the wonton, wild woman. Ritualized sex has a variety of differing pleasurable purposes, and can be practised to raise energy, to command magic or indeed to find a sense of spiritual communion with a partner or partners. All acts of love and pleasure can become rituals, sacramental acts of love.

In certain magical traditions, wanking and sexual release are common ways of raising magical energy and power. In her book *Natural Magic*, the prolific occult writer Doreen Valiente states that practitioners of sacred sex magic say that sex has three functions: propagation of the race, sheer enjoyment and revitalization by the exchange of vital magnetism. We must remember that this text was penned in 1975 and much has shifted since that date. Today, sacred and ritual sex is performed and celebrated by a multitude of witches and practitioners of the craft with differing sexualities and who have their own ideas about the "functions" of sex. Sexual experiences occur from the auto-sexual to multi-sexual, and we have seen a huge shift of "sexual labels" and definitions of sexuality in recent years.

However you approach it, the important thing in sex magic is to set an intention that you affirm before starting, that you wish to understand, connect or get to know yourself or your partner(s) more deeply.

The Passion Potion and flying ointment balm are perfect for application in sacred sexuality rituals, when people want to deepen their connection to each other and to the divine. The plant magic heightens the senses in such a way that gentle, considered touches can hold profound and mysterious meanings between lovers and spaces.

In sacred sex rites, application of the flying ointment and Passion Potion are best built up slowly in doses throughout the ritual. Flying ointment can be rubbed into the inner wrists and 13 drops of Passion Potion (depending on its strength) can be dripped into one another's mouths every half-hour or licked off the body. However, the balm is not to be ingested by mouth, so be aware of this.

EXPLORING YOUR OWN SEXUALITY

The realm of self-lust and self-pleasure is the perfect place to explore when becoming comfortable and accepting of your own sexual, sensual self. Through magical rites, you can create a personal space in which to investigate what it is that you actually like sexually, and what you need in order to feel safe and open. Potentially this is the place in which to ask yourself how you would like to communicate with another in sexual connection, and to find your own voice and ways to express your requests and desires.

Here follows a wonderful rite to help you connect with and explore your sexual nature, using the ointment. This self-pleasure ritual can be something you design and enjoy over the course of an entire day, flirting with the idea of taking yourself out and celebrating your sexuality, revelling in your sense of self care and love.

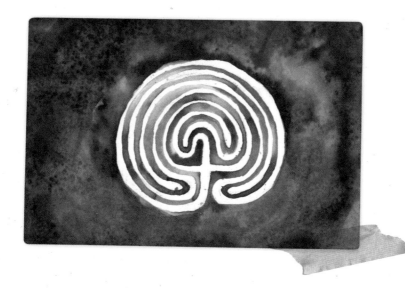

SELF-PLEASURE RITUAL

We will be calling on the powerful sensual seductress datura to hold this self-love rite, as the Divine Diva enables us to fall in lust with ourselves so beautifully. As the flowering seductress of the night, datura holds great powers to unleash our own seductress. She can facilitate a sexual awakening within ourselves.

Steps:

1. You can begin by creating and designing your own self-love altar. Perhaps place a picture of datura on the altar, and a chilli pepper or a mirror to symbolize self-love. Include symbols of all the other elements you wish to invite into your rite. Cast your circle for protection.

2. Now, set some intentions along the lines of:

   * raising your sexual energy
   * discovering what you enjoy most and what turns you on
   * exploring your own sexual power
   * staying in lust with yourself
   * working through anxieties around your body or sex
   * moving through shame

3. Then take a few drops of the passion potion, write out your intentions and set them on your altar.

4. Take some more drops of the Passion Potion and put on some suitable mood music. Plan some activities to enjoy next:

   * What makes your heart sing and your sexual organs tingle? Do it.
   * Get dressed in clothing, jewellery, make-up or shoes that make you feel attractive.
   * Take yourself out on a date, eat delicious food, indulge yourself.

5. If you receive any attention, hold your power, and know you are there for yourself, protected by those spikes from the datura seed pod.
6. When you return to your space, light a candle, sit facing your altar and read the following datura incantation:

Take me on a time-warp journey

Twisted labyrinth spiral bloom,

Maze walking ...

Singing the most sensual tune ...

Luminosity

Attracting night flyers,

Pollinate fertile creativity,

Inviting Venus,

Self-pleasure inducing

Temptress extreme.

Kali calling

Erotic attitude

Divinity

Many open faces,

Aspects flowing freely between,

The places seen and unseen ...

Empower shapeshifting sex magic,

Black, sharp-cornered seeds – imprint my DNA

In union with you own,

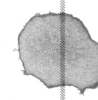

Distorted images becoming crystal-clear coaxing

Everlasting brain waves –

Excite, entice, allure

Slipping between tantalizing personalities.

7. Now clear your boudoir a little so the immediate area feels clear. Play some suitable relaxing or sensual music.
8. Burn your favourite incense and then disrobe. Relax and unwind.
9. Re-read your intention words before exploring your body.
10. Place a little of the flying ointment on your wrists and ankles, and start to self-massage, beginning with your face and head – giving thanks for your physical form for the ability to feel pleasure ...
11. Massage your neck and throat... arms ... chest ... torso ... buttocks.... anus... genitalia ... legs ... feet ...
12. Blow the candle out and whisper your thanks.

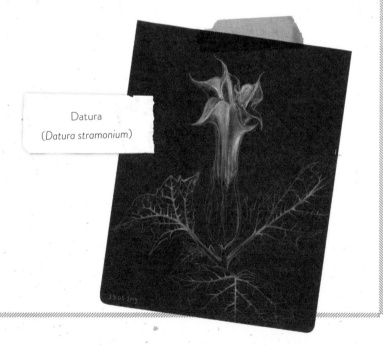

Datura
(*Datura stramonium*)

THE BALANCE OF OPPOSITES

Before we look at rituals for sex magic between couples, we want to clarify that when we talk about opposing forces – directive and receptive, straight and circular, yin and yang – we must remember that there is a constant nuanced dance between this seemingly dual aspect. We do not categorize ourselves as sexually straight or gay; we do not conform to what may be assigned to typically gendered traits and we are open to fluidity in all aspects of our magic, just as we are open to learning new perspectives in all aspects of our lives.

Opposing forces always have to consider the ever-present level of swirling, changing chaos that pervades in all our lives; perhaps this is an external force living outside duality. When considering a magic practice, the more we can become comfortable with the opposing forces within ourselves, the more we can embrace whatever challenges might arise. These might be challenges in our lives, or indeed created in the world, as we try to shift patterns or situations through the power of energy manipulation.

We need to be comfortable with the unknown, but we also might need a sense of purpose and a point to direct our energy toward. We need to be warm and open but courageous and have our boundaries strong, to find surrender but also strength, understanding but not collusion. We need to know ourselves – and we can learn so much about ourselves through working with the plants that often hold a mirror up to the things we haven't wanted to see in ourselves before. We love to work with nature's cycles to potentize all the work we do.

SACRED SEXUALITY

Sacred sexuality celebrates the power of inseparable but contradictory opposites; light and dark, receptive and directive, the yin and the yang. It was often written about these forces being represented by male and female, a misunderstood interpretation of the beauty of the fractal magic of polarities being contained within each other, whoever we are and identify as. One symbol used since time immemorial is the circle and the line, creating a binary code. We are now freer to explore more inclusive sex rites, to explore the non-binary and celebrate our differences.

A SACRED SEX RITE FOR COUPLES / MULTIPLES

Our beautiful witchy friend Sue describes the effects of sharing this next rite with her sacred lover, saying, "We have tried these methods with your balm previously – just walking in the woods and in sacred sexuality. Getting the dosage right was tricky to start with – I find I need more than him – but we both enjoy the tingle! As a magical couple practising sacred sexuality, it is easy to connect."

She continues: "Some of our friends who have tried the flying ointment only need a tiny bit in the crease of their elbows to feel the potency of the balm's transformative powers – some of them big men! It always surprises me how our tolerance levels differ."

Steps:

1. Choose a new moon and a time when you can focus and be in nature to begin experiences with the flying ointment balm.
2. Before you begin, create a spoken invocation or incantation to repeat to yourself three times on each application of the balm – write this down.
3. Create an altar space to potentize your balm – and place your written intention on your altar beside it.
4. Starting on your pulse points, rub in a little of the balm while repeating your mantra or intention to yourself three times. Observe your reactions.
5. Now take a walk in the wilds and ask the plants to guide you.
6. If you feel confident apply more balm to your skin or orifices – nostrils provide easy access. If using the balm vaginally or anally, be aware it is an oil-based recipe so if using condoms please check they are compatible.

EXPLORING THE POWER OF OPPOSITES

Writing in the 1970s, Doreen Valiente describes a beautiful sexual magical rite, which taps into the power of opposites by one person taking on contradictory yet complimentary energies, in this instance directive and receptive. Here is our adapted 21st-century rite ...

On a full moon night, two people are to perform a sacred dance around an oak tree. They begin by sitting facing one another and talking about what it is they wish to gain or create from this rite. They tell the oak tree.

Steps:

1. Both parties apply the hallucino-lube, the flying ointment, vaginally, anally or just a little on the pulse points. Then sitting in silence, they gaze into one another's eyes for a few moments.
2. Music can be played if desired for this next part. The person playing or feeling into the yin or receptive aspect of the couple gets up and begins a dance around the tree, followed by the person playing or feeling into the yang or directive aspect of the couple, who is in pursuit of them. Yin leads yang around and around and around, seven times around the oak – before yin lets yang catch hold of them properly and they exchange sexual energy, intercourse – communication with body, mind, spirit.
3. A leaf is chosen and taken from the tree (after asking its permission) and moistened with all the love-making secretions that have mingled inside the sexual cauldron of the body.
4. This leaf is a power talisman and may be carried to bring good fortune and accomplish their wishes for the rite.

- 17 -
FLYING TOWARD DEATH

he sands of time are moving through the hourglass continuously; we are all moving toward death. Yet living under the pressure of Grandfather Time, we are often too busy to pause and consider our place within the cycle of life and death.

"Why are we here?" and "what happens after we die?" are some of the biggest philosophical questions that can arise in our lives. Yet rushing through life leaves little space to practise being in the liminal state, and little time to dream and explore mystery and the unknown. So many people become scared of death. If, through life, we had the space to practise non-attachment and imagine death and dying, we potentially could live more fearlessly with increased joy, and have less anxiety when we arrive at the end of our life.

In our practices as clinical herbalists, we use our local herbal allies to support and aid in the shifting of perceptions, especially the fear and anxiety that can often surround a terminal diagnosis and impending death. Ideally, we should all learn to create rituals, and draw on medicines to support people's emotional and spiritual state as they walk toward their personal passing.

THE FEAR OF DEATH

If we look at the bigger picture, it seems clear that separating ourselves from death, which is a natural transition of the life cycle, is leading our society to the point of self-destruction. Our Western society's current paradigm, capitalism with its model of constant "growth", is fixed in the summer season. It is always moving and growing; never taking stock or stopping to decline, regroup and restore.

Interestingly, there has been an increased fear of death linked with technological advancements in medicine. As medicine has become more technological, our focus has been on preserving life at all costs for many years. People clearly at their end of life have been brought back to life to live incapacitated, unfulfilling lives, with immense pressure then placed on their families, emotionally and financially, to keep them properly cared for.

In recent years, there has been better professional support of the dying. However, our society remains disconnected from the realities of death itself, with little end-of-life care happening at home and families left feeling disempowered to help, not through a lack of wanting to provide care and support, but through a lack of experience with and disconnection from death generally in society. How many children even see dead animals, let alone grandparents or loved ones while they are near the end? In the race to advance medicine and prolong life, there are lasting effects on society as a whole that need to be addressed. Some steps have been taking in the recognition of this, but a broader reversal in this disconnection is long overdue.

Here in the West, we are raised in a culture where community rituals are often commercialized and turned into festivals of consumption, such as Easter, Halloween and Christmas. The general population grows up with a disconnect to nature. The chocolate binge that is now Easter is supposed to be a celebration of the Spring Equinox – a rebirth of the soil and the land after winter's colder, dormant times. Simply being outside and welcoming the new verdant growth of spring, observing nature's rhythms and celebrating with community was once the norm.

In the past, society marked and celebrated movement through the wheel of the year, feeling the cycle of life close by and witnessing it first-hand through the strong links to the land and seasons that farming and foraging mark.

In contemporary society, community rituals and happiness have so often been replaced with a sense of lack, and seeking of fulfilment. There is never enough – never enough gifts under the tree, enough food on the table, enough time, enough space, enough money. Addictions often manifest to mask feelings of lack and inadequacy. We find ourselves at a point in time where our addiction to consumption and hoarding wealth is destroying the very ecosystem we rely on for life.

APPROACHES TO DEATH

When someone with a terminal diagnosis seeks out a clinical herbalist, they come for their own personal reasons, but often people are searching for a way to survive. Hearing that we are going to die soon is scary and often induces a sense of panic. Feelings of shock and denial can arise after the diagnosis, and the resultant prognosis. This can then give rise to feelings of not being ready to accept or welcome death as part of the journey.

Many people fight hard for survival and the will to live can in certain circumstances override the death sentence given to them. Others have instinctive knowledge that although they're "not ready", they feel death knocking loudly, forcing them to come to terms with a shortened life span. We work with people to help them gently find the strength to face death.

We have explored using the flying ointment with people over the years in their approach toward accepting death and surrendering to the journey. Mugwort (*Artemisia vulgaris*) contained in the ointment is a birthing herb that strengthens uterine contractions. The herb also supports altered states of consciousness; a liminal space that, with practice, can release us from many of our fears and worries about embracing the unknown, whether in birth or in death. For most of human history, the process of birth has also been associated with death, and in many countries, that is still a reality. Those who have experienced birth have touched the brink between life and death. Childbirth is a threshold that brings danger for both baby and birthing parent. There are many postpartum rituals and expected or imposed confinement linked to traditions and religious practices that increase the capacity for rest and recuperation post-birth.

Holding a ritual naming circle to introduce the newborn to the Universe is a way to remember that children are not "ours"; not something we possess. They have separate destinies with their own reasons for being, and their own relationship, if they find one, to the sacred. A naming circle is a way to mark the baby's first passage between the worlds.

BIRTH AND DEATH

A report in 2020 found over two million pregnancies end in stillbirth globally. This intense grief brings with it a raging, painful storm that can leave whole families and communities devastated and paralysed with sadness. Creation and participation in a grief ritual can help to bring the grieving parents to a healing resolution.

There is a need for careful ceremony to bury miscarried, aborted and stillborn babies, to recognize the trauma and to give space to grieve. There is often little thought or attention given to this traumatic and extremely impactful time.

Health statistics in England show that one out of every eight recognized pregnancies ends in a miscarriage, with many more potentially occurring without the person knowing they are actually pregnant. Open communication and a general acknowledgement that support is needed for everyone involved would be helpful, given how common this experience is.

During miscarriage, flying ointment can be used to accept the inevitable and allow a graceful release of the foetus back to the Earth, wishing the spirit well and sending them off on their onward journey. Miscarriage is, however, still a taboo subject.

We are kept separate from much of the reality of childbirth, the experiences of the loss of babies, the blood. With medicalized hospital births, people sometimes meet their babies once they are dressed and cleaned, although this is becoming less common. There has been a recent boost in awareness of the benefits of skin-to-skin contact after birth and more support for parents who choose to breastfeed. However, there is much work to do in society as a whole concerning the awkwardness around conversations about death and loss. In our own practice, we like to invite the balm in as a gentle facilitator for exploring some of these themes.

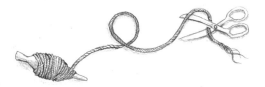

DREAMING DEATH

As we have seen, the flying ointment can be harnessed for dreaming practices. We can use dreaming techniques as tools with patients who are facing death. It is a space from which to explore ideas, subconscious patterns or beliefs, and unlock the sense of mystery greater than the self; the beginning of dissolving the ego. It can return us back to a state of new perception, like that we have within the womb or as a newborn. We can also use it to help us connect with other realms, as the oracles did of old.

ORACLES OF THE DEAD

Throughout time, humans have been fascinated with communications between the living and the dead, those entities in the spirit world who may have messages and insights for us or who need a little help in leaving the Earthly plane. Sometimes, people are motivated by the desires to send our respects and wishes to our ancestors, and ask for good graces in return.

Communication with the dead has been practised in a multitude of ways. Each culture across the globe has its own diverse rites and rituals surrounding the practice. There are plenty of morbid and macabre customs and procedures! A few involve using body parts, but most do not, and are more focused on simply contacting souls passed.

In the Caribbean a ritual called "nine nights" or "death yard" is observed where families and friends of the deceased come together to celebrate the person and to help their spirit move on, thus saving it from becoming restless. It is believed that the recent dead house their spirits for nine days and nights, in which time the spirit is called a "duppy", and if they are shown the correct customs and procedures they will not stay behind to haunt the living.

In the Hindu religion 13 days are observed for the death ritual to ensure the proper reincarnation of souls.

Old Norse literature writes of the chief deity singing the songs of the souls, as well as using "speech-runes" to "loosen the tongue" of the dead.

In more recent times, in the 1800s, séances were very *à la mode* all over Europe. The word séance comes from the French word for "session", from the

Old French *seoir*, "to sit". To sit in session involved chatting with the spirits. These sitting-in sessions happen today and are called "mediumship" in modern spiritualist churches. In personal oracle practice, and other spaces, this work is also called "necromancy". This sometimes confuses people into believing (incorrectly) that necrophilia is involved.

Necromancy has roots that go back millennia to the days when ancient shamans, witches and magicians first began to contact discarnate souls, summoning ghosts and questioning them on future events. The word "necromancy" translates as "divination by means of the dead", coming from the Greek *nekrosh* (dead) and *manteia* (divination). Some practitioners are fully conscious while functioning as contacts; others may slip into a partial or full trance, or into an altered state of consciousness. An invocation to henbane can open this work and is perfect to catalyse a descent to the underworld or other world realms, as we will see.

HENBANE'S RELATIONSHIP WITH DEATH

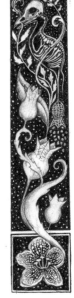

Guardian of the underworld, henbane has long been associated with death. Henbane is in the flying ointment, and is connected to the dark moon, crone energy and an association with the death rites of wakes and vigils. The herb aids folk to embrace and feel ready for their own death.

Henbane seeds have been found in a ritual Viking burial in Denmark. This inclusion of henbane could be evidence of her role as a seer, or to support her passing over into the realms beyond death.

Documented use of henbane in death rites goes back at least as far as the Neolithic period in Scotland. A Neolithic vessel showed evidence of henbane mixed with porridge, encrusted on the bowl fragments. The site of the find includes a timber enclosure. The bowl may have provided offerings to the dead, while the building acted as a mortuary to house the dead. This is potential evidence of magical, ritual belief in the flight of the spirit at the point of death.

FLYING TOWARD DEATH

THE USE OF HENBANE IN DEATH ACCEPTANCE

In our herbal clinical practice, we often spend time considering henbane and the folklore surrounding the plant with patients nearing the end of their life. We use the flying ointment with them to initiate gentle perceptive shifts, and then engage in creative writing, or discussion if the patient is too weak to write.

Concepts to explore in this way can include:

What are your personal fantasies surrounding death?
(For example, a Terry Pratchett fan told us that she had imagined her own Discworld and the Grim Reaper was always with her. They had a comic relationship, where she was forever telling him to hang on.)

Where do you imagine you might travel to?
(For example, heaven, hell, absorbed into the Universe, reincarnation, etc.)

Do you imagine you can still see and visit the living?
(Anxieties about who you will leave behind often arise. We often reach for henbane to alleviate these anxiety states.)

Who do you need to make peace with?

Who would you like to leave instructions or letters for?

How do you feel about leaving your physical body behind?

What plans would you have for a funeral?

How do you want to be remembered as an ancestor?

Can you see your descendants calling on you to support them? What can you offer them?
(Henbane can be used in an annual vigil for remembering the dead.)

INVOCATION TO HENBANE

Here follows an invocation to henbane to help us face death:

I call on you, Hades,

Raising a brew to Henbane,

Thundering Traveller journeying with death,

*Hold my pain in your jaws, bite the
agonies between your teeth –*

Ever rowing the river with my loved ones, lost ones

Soothing the waves

You, Transporter of Souls to the other world, the underworld

Taming the tremor,

Gift me the ability to laugh at life, to feel the joviality

Afterlife Apollo

Next level …

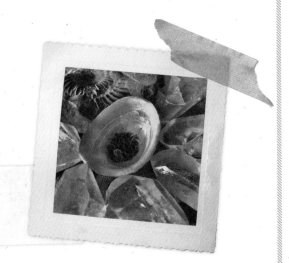

Henbane seeds
on the altar

THE STORY OF LIFE AND DEATH

Through story and connection to each other we can create supportive webs to hold us in our grief, bring joy where there is sadness and hope where there is despair.

The beautiful red and white toadstool, the fly agaric that holds the spell and story of this book, is the stuff of fairy tales, connecting us to a world of the imagination. It is linked with the quieter seasons in the natural world, popping up in late autumn and displaying themselves deep into the winter months – the death time of the cycle of the year. The toadstool and the mycelium beneath the floor of the forest, representations of the yarns of our lives, are powerful instruments in exploring death and dying.

Vibrant community rituals, festivals and storytelling during our lifetime creates space where we can dream and imagine places that are outside of the familiar. This can ease us toward being comfortable with the unknown.

When, through our herbal practice, we support people facing their death, our work connects them with their past and their stories. Herbs can guide them to look forward, beyond death, to a place that is unknown, but perhaps becomes better prepared for. There is a sense through this work that if an individual feels held, heard and supported in their death, there can be less fear around surrendering to it.

Storytelling helps us make sense of our environment and personal experiences. Many of our older stories are traditional folktales. They represent the richness of oral patterns of telling, and are the product of a community experience. When we log people's lives through their stories, we gather the vessels with which we can remember and celebrate their life far beyond death.

Gifts of winter solstice have been misconstrued – now adding to the decline of life through consumerism. Driven by an urge to "please" and "gift" family and friends, people are sucked into buying stuff every Christmas, a holiday ripe with imagery of pine trees, toadstools in the form of "Father Christmas", and birth of new life, with the winter solstice and the return of the sun.

This toadstool offers the ability to fly, to journey high above the plane we normally inhabit. This mushroom allows us to take the eagle's view with the ability to move away from social pressures and forge a new path. What better gift can we give each other and our culture that to revive and re-story ritual and remembrance with our local plants? To rebuild community and support one another as our species spins on a trajectory of consumption, we have the power to create new myth and story – and fly agaric holds some of those keys.

When there are stories of fear and pain and terror, we can transmute those stories with the herbs and connect with the Saturn energy, the death energy and Grandfather Time.

More importantly, how can we learn to accept the inevitable end of physical life when we have become so disconnected from death and the dying, even from death within the animal world for sourcing meat?

The planet will survive and adapt, but can our species survive? Can we change the narrative, embracing death once more and bringing the stories of death back into our culture? We need to practise accepting the mystery, touching the void, releasing fear, facing our demons and also the overwhelming beauty of life. We can prepare for the inevitable challenges that we face as we move on as individuals or as a species. The flying ointment and this family of witching herbs can support this journey. For they themselves represent our own internal fears and those we share as a collective society.

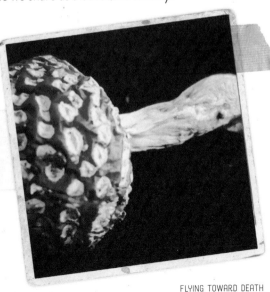

Fly Agaric
(Amanita muscaria)

EPILOGUE
TOUCHING MYSTERY

s you have discovered, we Seed Sistas love all plants, especially the medicinal herbs that we draw on time and time again for our own health, the health of our families and the health of our communities. We are passionately potty about plants – and the ones which gave us permission to be truly wild are the witching herbs. To them we owe a ginormous debt.

It is indeed a mysterious adventure that we all walk with these wonderful witching herbs, these beauties enlighten us about the space where magic and medicine mingle, where 21st-century science and ancient craft touch. Prolonged ill health and disease, be it mental, physical, emotional or spiritual, can be accompanied by *seeking* a connection to something "other", something "bigger" than ourselves to alleviate discomfort and give meaning to our very existences. We celebrate the places where these plant guides lead us on a familiar journey inside ourselves, a re-remembering of times gone by. These herbs are multifaceted; they can heal physical ails, be used for recreational purposes – for restoration, for play and for imaginative magic.

The witching herbs aid and support our relationship with nature, to other beings and to humankind. Impactful teachers, they demand respect and we need to understand our own boundaries and hone our skills of perception in relation to them.

Fear perpetuates society these days and there are huge amounts of fear directed at these plants, the so-called poisons – the witching herbs. Fear of the counter-culture, the fear of medics and the fear of herbalists are the result of society having divided things into binary sections: poison or medicine, helpful or dangerous. As we have seen, these plants are nuanced with the potential

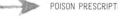

for formidable, fast-acting physical effects and more subtle energetic effects depending on the dose and method in which they are taken.

They counsel to approach with clear intent. Come to meet them gently, draw them, grow them, connect with them. Create witching herb gardens and watch the magic grow. Teach our children and communities not to eat the flowers or berries of these plants, as we do when teaching them about foxgloves and hemlock. We cannot rid the Earth of these things we fear just because we have misunderstood them. Instead, let's celebrate the opportunities for healing our relationship with nature.

In these pages we have shared the ways in which the witching herbs have been the catalyst for bringing magic into our clinical practices as herbalists, and also into our lives more generally. You cannot deny a sense of magic when you work closely with these powerful beings.

The power herbs have many amazing physical actions that we need to know how to draw on in clinical practice with patients. However, we also need to look beyond the actions elicited by the botanical chemistry, to see what these herbs have to offer us on other levels. This is particularly relevant in today's world, where psycho-emotional health issues – referred to in society as mental illness – are so prevalent, especially among young people.

A renaissance of these herbs could create a sense of connectedness and put ritual back into working with plants. We have experienced universal oneness and the interconnectedness of all of life through growing and imbibing these herbs, tapping into a sense of both timelessness and time travel.

These plants have stories to share and gifts of insight to offer, allowing us to access ecstatic states, channelling Aphrodite, like the raving ones, the Maenads of the Bacchanalia. Creating the flying ointment has certainly enabled us to draw on that energy and be swept away under their Solanaceae enchantment.

We have shared with you the ethereal, mythical potential of each herb, their clinical applications and their emotional effects. We love these plants deeply and hope we have conveyed our sentiments about their absolute *golden* qualities!

It is time to accept that there are many valid ways to research plants. If we each create journals reflecting on our interactions with plants, we can build up a body of work that explores and collates information, supporting each other in our learning and connection. Creative ways of depicting our experiences with the plants will help to keep their spirits alive and pass on their knowledge in accessible ways.

We call on the whole global herbal community, plant lovers everywhere, to embrace these plants again. Note down what you see and how you work with them. Create magical rituals with your communities, instil a sense of wonder in the natural world with all that come into contact with you.

We call on you to grow these herbs and learn about them, educate others.

We call on all the travellers to other states of consciousness to tread wisely with these herbs, draw them, grow them and work with them so that you truly know them. Enter into sacred relationship.

May these words carry into your hearts the resonance that the witching herbs have gifted to us of pure magic, powerful medicine and a message of hope and possibility.

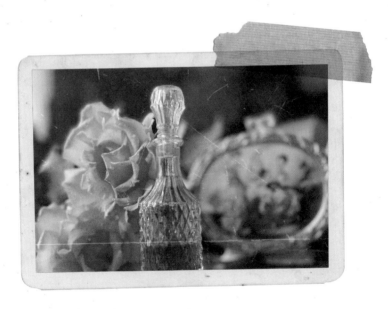

BIBLIOGRAPHY

Alizadeh, A., Moshiri, M., Alizadeh, J., Balali-Mood, M. (2014). Black henbane and its toxicity – a descriptive review. In: *Avicenna Journal of Phytomedicine* [Internet]. 4(5), 297–311. Available from: www.ncbi.nlm.nih.gov/pmc/articles/PMC4224707/

Aldred, L. (2000). Plastic Shamans and Astroturf Sun Dances: New Age Commercialization of Native American Spirituality. In: *The American Indian Quarterly*, Lincoln: University of Nebraska Press. 24(3): 329–352

Anadón, A., Aránzazu Martínez, M. (2016). *Nutraceuticals Efficacy, Safety and Toxicity*. London: Academic Press, pp. 855–874

Baker, E. W. (2016). The Salem Witch Trials. In: *Oxford Research Encyclopaedias*. Available at: oxfordre.com/americanhistory/view/10.1093/acrefore/9780199329175.001.0001/acrefore-9780199329175-e-324

Baker, J. R. (1994). The Old Woman and Her Gifts: Pharmacological Bases of the Chumash use of Datura. In: *Curare*, 17(2): 253–276

Baker, M. (2011). *Discovering the Folklore of Plants*, 3rd edition, Oxford: Shire Classics

Behringer, W. (2004). *Witches and Witch-Hunts: A Global History*. Cambridge: Polity Press

Bevan-Jones, R. (2009). *Poisonous Plants: A Cultural and Social History*. Oxford: Windgather Press

Busia, K., Heckels, F. (2006). Jimson Weed: History, Perceptions, Traditional Uses, and Potential Therapeutic Benefits of the Genus Datura. In: *HerbalGram*, 69: 40–50

Callaway, C. (1970). *The religious system of the AmaZulu*. Cape Town: Struik

Carter, A. J., (1996). Narcosis and Nightshade. In: *BMJ*. Vol. 313 (7072): 1630–1632. doi: 10.1136/bmj.313.7072.1630

Chevalier A. (1996). Mandragora officinarum. In: *Encyclopaedia of Medicinal Plants*. London: Dorling Kindersley, p. 230

Davis, Wade. (2000). *Passage of Darkness: The Ethnobiology of the Haitian Zombie*. Chapel Hill: University of North Carolina Press=

Dormandy, T. (2012). *Opium: Reality's Dark Dream*. New Haven: Yale University Press

Friend, Hilderic. *Flower Lore*. Rockport, MA: Para Research, 1981

Gilani, A. H., Khan, A. U., Raoof, M., Ghayur, M. N., Siddiqui, B. S., Vohra, W., Begum, S. (2008). Gastrointestinal, selective airways and urinary bladder relaxant effects of Hyoscyamus niger are mediated through dual blockade of muscarinic receptors and Ca2+ channels. At: *Fundamental & clinical pharmacology* [Internet]; 22(1): 87–99. Available from: onlinelibrary.wiley.com/doi/10.1111/j.1472-8206.2007.00561.x/full

289

Gillam, Frederick. (2008). *Poisonous Plants in Great Britain.* Glastonbury: Wooden Books

Goodyear, John (trans.) and Robert T. Gunther (ed); (1655/1934). *The Greek Herbal of Dioscorides.* Oxford: Oxford University Press

Greenaway, K. (1884, 2015). *The Language of Flowers.* Alchester: Pook Press

Haller, Jr, J. S. (1984). Aconite: A Case Study in Doctrinal Conflict and the Meaning of Scientific Medicine. *Bulletin of the New York Academy of Medicine.* 60: 888–904

Hansen, Harold A., (1983). *The Witch's Garden.* York Beach: Samuel Weiser

Harrod Buhner, S., (1998). *Sacred and Herbal Healing Beers.* Boulder: Brewers Publications

Hastis, T., (2015). *Witches' Ointment: The Secret History of Psychedelic Magic.* Rochester, VT: Park Street Press

Hermann, P., Mitchell, S. A. and Jens Peter Schjødt, J. P. and Rose, A. J., ed. (2017). *Old Norse Mythology: Comparative Perspectives.* Cambridge, MA: Harvard University Press

History.com Editors .(2017, 2020). History of Witches. History website. Available at: www.history.com/topics/folklore/history-of-witches

Hobson, G. (1978). The Rise of the White Shaman as a New Version of Cultural Imperialism. In: Hobson, G., ed. *The Remembered Earth.* Albuquerque, NM: Red Earth Press, 100–108

Hort, A. (trans). (1926). *Theophrastus: Enquiry into Plants.* Cambridge, MA: Loeb Classical Library

Hyslop, J., and Ratcliffe, P. (1989). *A Folk Herbal.* Oxford: Radiation

Höfler, M. (1908). *Volksmedizinische Botanik Der Germanen.* Vienna: Ludwig

Jahn, S., Seiwert, B., Kretzing, S., Abraham, G., Regenthal, R., Karst, U. (2012). Metabolic studies of the Amaryllidaceous alkaloids galantamine and lycorine based on electrochemical simulation in addition to in vivo and in vitro models. In: *Anal Chim Acta.* 756: 60–72. doi: 10.1016/j.aca.2012.10.042. Epub 1 Nov 2012.

Jiménez-Mejías, M. E., Montaño-Díaz, M., López Pardo, F., Campos Jiménez, E.;

Moldenke, Harold N. and Alma L. Moldenke. (1952). *Plants of the Bible.* New York, NY: The Ronald Press Company

Jones, A. (1995). Case Study: The European Witch Hunts, c. 1450–1750 and Witch Hunts Today. Gendercide Watch website.

Kanner, L. (1935). *Folklore of the Teeth.* New York: MacMillan

Kellett, C., (2009). *Poison and Poisoning: A Compendium of Cases, Catastrophes and Crimes.* Cardiff: Accent Press

Kluckhohn, C. (1944:2). *Navaho Witchcraft.* Boston: Beacon Press

Lambers, H., Chapin, F. S., Pons, T. L. (2008). Ecological biochemistry: allelopathy and defense against herbivores. In: *Plant Physiology Ecology.* New York, NY: Springer. pp. 445–77

Lehner, E. and Lehner, J. (1960, 2003). *Folklore and Symbolism of Flowers, Plants and Trees*, New York: Dover

Lewis, W. H. and Elvin, Lewis, M. P. F. (2003). *Medical Botany: Plants Affecting Human Health*. Second edition, Hoboken, NJ: John Wiley & Sons

Li, H. (1977). Hallucinogenic Plants in Chinese Herbals. In: *Botanical Museum Leaflets*. Cambridge, MA: Harvard University. 25 (6): 161–181

Lin, C. C., Chan, T. Y. and Deng, J. F. (2004). Clinical Features and Management of Herb-Induced Aconitine Poisoning. In: *Annals of Emergency Medicine*. 43: 574–579

Lilienfeld, S. (2002). Galantamine: a novel cholinergic drug with a unique dual mode of action for the treatment of patients with Alzheimer's disease. In: *CNS Drug Rev*. Summer; 8(2): 159–76

MacCoitir, N. (2015). *Ireland's Wild Plants – Myths, Legends & Folklore*. Cork: Collins Press

Mann, J. (2000). *Murder, magic, and medicine*. New York, NY: Oxford University Press

Martín Cordero, M. C., Ayuso González, M. J. and González de la Puente, M. A. (1990). Intoxicación atropínica por Mandragora autumnalis: descripción de quince casos [Atropine poisoning by Mandragora autumnalis: a report of 15 cases]. In: *Medicina Clínica*. 95 (18): 689–92

Mitchell, S., (2017). Óðinn, Charms and Necromancy: Hávamál 157 in its Nordic and European Contexts. In: *Old Norse Mythology – Comparative Perspectives*. Cambridge, MA: Harvard University Press, pp. 289–321

Netter, M. W. (1888). The "Mandrake" Medical Superstition. In: *The Medical Standard*. Vol. III. Chicago: G.P. Englehard. 173–75

Oldfather, C. H. (trans). (1935). *Diodorus of Sicily*. Cambridge, MA: Loeb Classical Library

Ott, J., Hofmann, A., (1993). *Pharmacotheon: Entheogenic Drugs, Their Plant Sources and History*. Natural Products Company

Paulsen, B. S. (2010). Highlights through the history of plant medicine. In: *Norwegian Academy of Science and Letters* [Internet]. Available at: www.dnva.no/binfil/download.php?tid=48677

Palmer, T. R. (1974). An Examination of Navaho Witchcraft and its Influence on the Thoughts and Actions of the Navaho People. In: *All Graduate Plan B and other Reports*. Utah State University. 945. Available at: digitalcommons.usu.edu/gradreports/945

von Perger, K. R. (1864). *Deutsche Pflanzensagen*. Stuttgart and Oehringen: Schaber

Piomelli, D. and Pollio, A. (1994). In upupa o stripe. A Study in Renaissance Psychotropic Plant Ointments. In: *Hist. Phil. Life Sci*. 16: 241–73

Ramoutsaki, I. A., Askitopoulou, H., Konsolaki, E. (2002). Pain relief and sedation in Roman Byzantine texts: Mandragoras officinarum, Hyoscyamos niger, and Atropa belladonna. In: *International Congress Series* [Internet]. Vol. 1242: 43–50. Available at: dx.doi.org/10.1016/S0531-5131(02)00699-4

Ratsch, C. (2005). *The Encyclopedia of Psychoactive Plants Ethnopharmacology and Its Applications*. Rochester, VT: Park Street

Ratsch, C., Dieter-Storl, W., and Muller-Ebeling, C. (2003). *Witchcraft Medicine: Healing Arts, Shamanic Practices, and Forbidden Plants*. Rochester, VT: Inner Traditions – Bear and Company

Raedisch, L. (2011). *Night of the Witches: Folklore, Traditions & Recipes for Celebrating Walpurgis Night*. Woodbury, MN: Llewellyn Publications

Roth, H. (2017). *The Witching Herbs: 13 Essential Plants and Herbs for Your Magical Garden*. Newbury Port, MA: Red Wheel/Weiser

Russel, J. B. (1984). *A History of Heaven: Witchcraft in the Middle Ages*. Ithaca, NY: Cornell University Press

Sengupta, T., Vinayagam, J., Nagashayana, N. et al. (2011). Antiparkinsonian effects of aqueous methanolic extract of *Hyoscyamus niger* seeds result from its monoamine oxidase inhibitory and hydroxyl radical scavenging potency. In: *Neurochem Res*. [Internet]. 36: 177. Available at: link.springer.com/article/10.1007/s11064-010-0289-x

Safford, W. E. (1920). Daturas of the Old World and New: An account of their narcotic properties and their use in oracular and initiatory ceremonies. In: *Smithsonian Report*. 2644: 537–67

Simpson, J. and Roud, S. (2000). *A Dictionary of English Folklore*, Oxford: Oxford University Press

Singh, V. (2017). Sushrata: The father of surgery. In: *Natl J Maxillofac Surg*. Jan–Jun; 8(1): 1–3. Available at: www.ncbi.nlm.nih.gov/pmc/articles/PMC5512402/ doi: 10.4103/njms.NJMS_33_17

Stewart, A. (2010). *Wicked Plants: The A–Z of Plants that kill, maim, intoxicate and otherwise offend*. London: Timber Press

Storms, G. (1948). *Anglo Saxon Magic* (PDF hosted at the Radboud Repository of the Radboud University Nijmegen)

Thompson, C. J. S. (1934). The Mandrake and the gallows legend. In: *ancient Greece*. London: Rider and Co. pp. 165–77

de Vries, H. (1993). Heilige bäume, bilsenkraut und bildzeitung. In *Naturverehrung und Heilkunst*, ed. C. Raetsch: Suedergellersen, Germany: Verlag Bruno Martin, pp. 65–83

INTERNET RESOURCES

www.academia.edu/40070517/Sagas_of_the_Solanaceae_Speculative_ethnobotanical_perspectives_on_the_Norse_berserkers

www.atlasobscura.com/foods/toloache-datura-innoxia

www.britishhomeopathic.org

data.unicef.org/resources/a-neglected-tragedy-stillbirth-estimates-report/

doctorlib.info/herbal/encyclopedia-psychoactive-plants-ethnopharmacology/56.html

en.natmus.dk/historical-knowledge/denmark/prehistoric-period-until-1050-ad/the-viking-age/religion-magic-death-and-rituals/a-seeress-from-fyrkat/

erenow.net/ancient/greek-fire-poison-arrows-scorpion-bombs/5.php

www.fragrantica.com/news/DATURA-3205.html

www.gardenorganic.org.uk/sites/www.gardenorganic.org.uk/files/organic-weeds/datura-stramonium.pdf

www.gutenberg.org/files/53202/53202-h/53202-h.htm

hekatecovenant.com/resources/symbols-of-hekate/crossroads/

hightimes.com/culture/flashback-friday-jimsonweed-the-worlds-worst-dope/

www.icysedgwick.com/necromancy/

en.wikipedia.org/wiki/Mandrake_the_Magician

nah.sen.es/vmfiles/abstract/NAHV1N1201328_38EN.pdf

naturemeetsculturestories.wordpress.com/2016/10/17/datura-thorny-history/

www.ncbi.nlm.nih.gov/pmc/articles/PMC2359130/pdf/bmj00573-0066.pdf

www.ncbi.nlm.nih.gov/pmc/articles/PMC539425/

www.theplantlist.org/browse/A/Solanaceae/Atropa/

pointshistory.com/2020/01/07/magic-cures-and-their-discontents-the-belladonna-treatment-in-the-early-twentieth-century/

www.rcpe.ac.uk/sites/default/files/w_lee_2.pdf

sciencenorway.no/drugs-history-plants/crazed-viking-warriors-may-have-been-high-on-henbane/1571431

INDEX

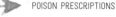

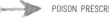

ALSO BY THE SEED SISTAS

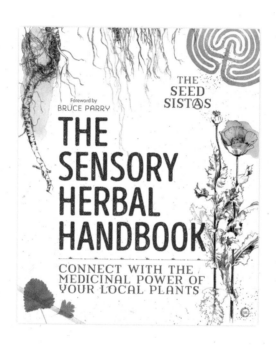

The Sensory Herbal Handbook
ISBN: 978-178678-211-3 (Paperback)
ISBN: 978-178678-261-8 (eBook)
ISBN: 978-178678-584-8 (Audio)

GRATITUDES

We are blessed with a strong community of plant lovers and there were a host of wonderful, supportive creatives who offered their time and expertise toward the writing of this book.

Our gratitude goes to:

Katie Shellard and Sue Ealding for the very first eyes and edits; Sue for sex magic consultations; Hannah Marsh for meticulous proofreading and wise input; Melinda McDougall for care and help with the structure and flow of our words; Ali Yellop for offering insightful suggestions; Anneliese (Primrose) Lambeth-Mansell and our own Kristin (Fennel) Walker for their opened eyes on the sex chapter; Nick Rowley for his encouragement and never-ending kindness; Adam Gordon for his support and help; Fiona Robertson, our fabulous editor and champion; and Mike Heckels, for their thorough grammar corrections. All the herbalists whose input and preparation suggestions we have featured: Katherine Bellchambers-Wilson, Geoffrey Dorje Soma, Latifa Pelletier-Ahmed, Jean Dow, Anne Cheshire and Christopher Hedley. Vic, for the fabulous and hilarious input with giant integrity on brewing. Our family members for your unwavering support. Hazza, Mars, Ziggy-May and Ash for coming along on this wild ride with us and for all the lessons you bring – we love you lot.

Silva, the illustrator, would like to thank her amazing family and friends for their support and the most incredible creator Mother Earth.

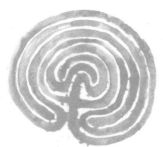

INDEX ◀

ABOUT THE AUTHORS

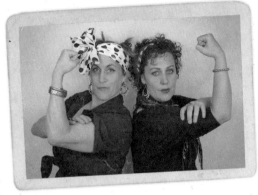

Kazz Goodweather (formally known as Karen Lawton) and Fiona Heckels are the Seed Sistas. They are hedge witches, authors, public speakers, clinical herbalists and eco-activists, and are passionate about sharing the magic of plant medicine education. Their first book, *The Sensory Herbal Handbook*, is a popular guide to getting to know your local plants through medicine, art, poetry and magic.

Their mission is to redefine what it means to be successful and to build resilient, thriving, communities that care deeply for their local green spaces. They meld clinical experience with ritual, art and creativity to teach herbalism in a unique, motivating and accessible style. They allow the plants to guide them to ever more ridiculous productions, passing on knowledge about herbs as home remedies to all who will listen, weaving spells of inspiration for creative activism.

ABOUT THE ILLUSTRATOR

Silva de Majo is an artist, sensory herbalist and horticulturist. Her work draws from a lifetime of observation and experience living closely with nature across the UK, where she has become known for her prodigious talent and an artistic approach that weaves the scientific with the mystical.

Her work reflects the interconnected web of life and has appeared on every surface imaginable from skin to ceramics, festival floats and gallery wall. Inspired by her surroundings, ideas and energy from nature, Silva forages the plants, seeds, fungi, earth, metals and minerals used to fabricate the materials and mediums for her alchemical and botanical works.

Like some of the plants that feature in this book, Silva lives on the edge of a field, blossoming in a creative network, with roots deep in the creative arts and in her garden.